TRAVEL HEALTH GUIDE

Everything You Need to Know Before You Leave, While You're Away, After You're Back

DR. MARK WISE

FIREFLY BOOKS

CONTENTS

INTRODUCTION

The purpose of this book is not to alarm you about all sorts of exotic infections and weird and scary conditions. Most people going to most places are fine most of the time. But it is important to be aware of the risks involved in travel, to know how to minimize those risks, and to know what to do if adversity or problems arise.

I practice Family Medicine and Travel and Tropical Medicine. I have served as the medical advisor to some outstanding organizations such as CUSO-VSO, Right To Play, Canadian Crossroads International, Free The Children and Engineers Without Borders. It has also been my honor to help prepare Canadian peacekeepers on their way to Afghanistan, as well as countless others who travel for humanitarian reasons. I continue to learn from my travelers, not just about travel-related illnesses, but more importantly, about different cultures, religions, traditions and the myriad reasons why people choose to travel. This is what makes my job so interesting and rewarding. I remain the world's most vicarious traveler.

However, not all of my travels have been vicarious. Over the past several years, as Chairman of the Board of Canadian Feed The Children, I have accompanied volunteers to Bolivia and Ethiopia to witness the worthwhile work we do support, and to see two amazing countries. All of my children have now traveled abroad once or twice with me, and my goal now is to do the same with my lovely granddaughter, Hannah, and any other grandchildren who might appear in the future!

There have been many changes in the field of travel medicine in the last decade including new and improved vaccines and medications against infections. Climate, geography, economics and politics continue to affect where people travel and why. And as along as poverty persists, there will always be a need for travelers to take precautions and care.

The following is a summary of the points I will emphasize in the coming pages:

- Use your common sense. It's the most important thing you can take along with you.
- Be proactive about your health. Stay physically and mentally fit, well rested and well fed.
- Get the recommended and/or required pre-travel inoculations. Visit a travel clinic.
- The most common problems will be related to your stomach and bowels. So remember to *boil it, bottle it, filter it, purify it, peel it, cook it … or forget it.*
- Take along something to treat diarrhea.
- Carry the appropriate medications and medical supplies.
- Avoid mosquitoes and other insects. Use an effective insect repellent such as DEET — day and night. In malarious areas, sleep under a mosquito net.
- Don't believe everything you hear or read about malaria and antimalarial drugs. But please believe what you read in this book. Take your antimalarial medication as directed.
- HIV/AIDS is transmitted through blood, blood products and unprotected sex. Abstain from casual sex, or use a latex condom — every time.
- Avoid driving in rural areas after dark. Beware of motorbikes and wear a searbelt.
- Be aware of your personal safety at all times. Carry adequate medical and travel insurance.

I sincerely hope that you find this book enjoyable and useful, and may all of your travels, regardless of the destination or purpose, be fulfilling and healthy.

PART 1

BEFORE YOU LEAVE

Chapter 1

BEFORE YOU LEAVE

Once you have decided to go away, whether for a week or for two years, the fun begins. In any case, you will undoubtedly have many things on your mind, such as planning your itinerary, preparing a budget, deciding what to pack, getting to the airport on time — and much more. One of the items on your list should be your health while you are abroad. So you should ask yourself some questions:

- Do I need any inoculations or shots before I go?
- Will I be traveling in areas that have malaria?
- What medications and supplies should I take along?
- Are there any safety precautions I should be aware of?
- I may be pregnant. Is that OK?
- What will I do for clean water?
- What do I do and who do I see if I become sick while I'm away?
- If something's wrong with me when I get home, who's going to figure that out?

Now that you've asked yourself all these questions, you should arrange to see your doctor. If he or she isn't able to provide the accurate, up-to-date advice you need, then you should probably head off to see someone at a travel clinic. Whether it's a doctor or a nurse, this someone should know a great deal about travel medicine.

Your travel medicine professional needs to know about general medicine, as patients will be of all ages and with all sorts of medical problems. He or she needs to be aware of the infectious and non-infectious health risks associated with traveling abroad. And he or she needs some insight into human behavior — why people travel and what they do when they are away. Knowledge of geography, politics, religion and history also come in handy. Hopefully your travel advisor will have a few masks or foreign photos on his walls, suggesting he or she is an experienced traveler and has actually been to some of the same places as you.

A travel medicine professional can advise you about vaccines, antimalarials and precautions, but remember *the doctor advises ... the patient decides*. So, you should base your decisions upon several factors, such as your perception of the risks, your love of needles and your budget.

However, pre-travel advice should be about much more than just needles and pills. You should also learn how your own personal behavior can greatly lessen the likelihood of most infections and other misfortunes. As well, you should find out how to deal with certain medical problems, should they arise.

When people start to plan their more exotic, or even not so exotic trips, one of the first things that enters their minds is *"What shots will I need?"* The answer to this seemingly simple question is not always so clear, nor is there always just one answer. But in general, it is all about the *risk*. And assessing that risk requires knowledge of geography, medicine and human behavior.

Vaccines are, in my opinion, one of the miracles of modern medicine. With a small, albeit possibly painful and relatively inexpensive injection in the arm, and almost no change in behavior, you will receive very good, or virtually perfect protection from an infection that has killed and continues to kill children and adults around the world. If we also had vaccines against HIV/AIDS, TB and malaria, what a difference it would make.

As I will repeat several times over the course of this book, risk may depend upon several factors such as:

13

- **Destination(s)** — An important factor, but far from the only one.
- **Duration of travel** — The longer you are away and exposed to certain conditions, the greater your risk.
- **Purpose of travel** — Certain activities, such as overseas medical work or volunteering in a small community, will be riskier than sitting behind a desk or sightseeing.
- **Style of travel** — The budget traveler or the VFR (Visiting Friends and Relatives – see Special Travelers) will have greater exposure than the businessperson who rarely leaves his or her five-star hotel.
- **Age** — Certain age groups may be more (or less) susceptible to certain infections, or have riskier behaviors.

- **Time of year** — Some infections such as dengue, malaria, meningitis and Japanese encephalitis may be seasonal in certain places.
- **Urban vs. rural** — Some infections might be a greater risk in rural areas due to the nature of the vector or the degree of poverty.
- **Other medical conditions or medications** — HIV/AIDS, allergies, diabetes, pregnancy and preexisting immunity might all influence the choice of vaccines; the likelihood of adverse effects and/or the effectiveness of the vaccine may vary with age.
- **Cost** — As vaccines can be costly and may be beyond the budget of many, it is often necessary to prioritize.
- **Personal preference** — In consultation with a travel medicine professional, you will decide which vaccines are right for you.

So to illustrate: Mr. and Mrs. Low Risk Traveler may be taking a ten-day cruise through Vietnam, Malaysia and Thailand, stopping only for daytime visits in the various ports. All of their meals and medical care are available on board. But Mr. and Mrs. High Risk Traveler will be volunteering for one year in a refugee camp along the Thai-Cambodian border. As I'm sure you'll agree, the approaches to these two types of travelers might be a bit different!

We divide all available vaccines into:

- **ROUTINE** — Everyone, traveling or not, should be up to date with these.
- **REQUIRED** — Proof of vaccination will be needed to enter certain countries or to cross certain international borders.
- **RECOMMENDED** — These should be given according to your risk, as outlined above.

The following provides a brief description of the vaccine-preventable infections and their vaccines. Please refer to table on page 34 for more details.

ROUTINE VACCINATIONS

Tetanus - diphtheria - pertussis - polio — Although these infections have largely been eliminated in most industrialized countries, they continue to be a risk for certain travelers. Despite great efforts, polio still exists in a handful of countries, including Nigeria, Egypt, India, Pakistan, Niger and Afghanistan. Tetanus, also known as lockjaw, can be a risk anywhere from a contaminated puncture wound. Most children are up-to-date with these vaccines. Adults should receive tetanus-diphtheria every 10 years, and a one-time polio booster if they are at risk of exposure.

Measles - mumps - rubella — Measles in particular continues to be a major killer among children in less developed countries. This is a "live" vaccine that should be avoided in pregnancy. It is routinely given after the first birthday, with a second dose before the age of 5 to provide lifelong immunity. Those born between 1957 and 1980 in the U.S., and between 1970 and 1980 in Canada, should receive a second dose if they have not previously done so. Infants between six months and a year who are traveling to an area of risk (e.g., Africa) should receive one dose of the vaccine, and will still need two further doses after the age of one.

Varicella (chicken pox) — Many adults acquired this infection when they were younger and are immune. Children routinely receive this vaccine now. Adults or children with no history of this viral infection may consider vaccination. This is a "live" vaccine and should not be given during pregnancy or to the immunosuppressed.

Pneumococcal pneumonia — Children routinely receive vaccination against this in childhood. Adults over the age of 65, or those with underlying medical problems such as heart and lung disease, diabetes, sickle cell disease and those without a spleen should receive a dose of Pneumovax®.

Influenza — This is an unpleasant viral infection passed through coughing and sneezing and close personal contact. It should not be confused with the common cold, which is a much milder viral illness. The symptoms of influenza include chills, fever, sore throat, muscle pains, severe headaches, diarrhea, coughing and weakness.

In the usual seasonal outbreaks, the elderly and those with underlying medical problems are the most vulnerable. The pandemic of H1N1 (swine flu), which first appeared in Mexico in April 2009, has been more serious in healthy young children and adults and pregnant women. Bird flu, caused by the H1N5 virus, has been responsible for deaths in Asia but has not spread worldwide as feared. The northern and southern hemispheres experience influenza outbreaks at opposite times of the year. Between lineups at airports and crowded planes and ships, travelers are exposed to lots of sneezing and coughing people!

Handwashing is an important line of defense against influenza, and masks may be worn if you are at high risk of exposure. If in Asia, refrain from handling live poultry. The mainstay of prevention, however, is vaccination. As I write this, two vaccines, one for the usual seasonal flu and one for H1N1, are being given. Influenza vaccines should not be given to people allergic to eggs. Side effects are usually mild and you will not develop "the flu" from the vaccine. Influenza vaccine provides protection only for the coming "season," as the responsible viruses tend to change from year to year.

Influenza, whether presumptive or laboratory proven, is usually treated with supportive measures: fluids, rest and acetaminophen (and chicken soup!). Antivirals, such as osel-tamivir (Tamiflu®) or zanamivir (Relenza®), may be used to shorten the duration of the illness or to treat the more susceptible or sicker individuals.

REQUIRED VACCINATIONS

Yellow fever — Yellow fever (YF) is a serious mosquito-borne viral infection which occurs in parts of South America and Africa (see maps on following page). It is transmitted by the *Aedes aegypti* mosquito, which can be found in both urban and rural areas. It tends to occur in outbreaks or epidemics rather than being "endemic." It is a very serious infection, which begins as a flu-like illness with fever, headache, nausea, loss of appetite and muscle pains. In some, this progresses to jaundice (yellowing of the skin and eyes), liver failure and hemorrhage. There is no specific treatment available, and mortality rates are at least 20 percent. While rare in travelers, perhaps because most people are immunized, it is still a risk even for that short cruise down the Amazon.

Other than meningococcal vaccine as described below, YF vaccine is the only one that may be required (not just recommended) for international travel. A certificate of vaccination must be shown to get a visa or enter certain countries. Many cruise lines will not allow you on board unless you have the certificate (even sometimes when it is not needed). The rules are as follows:

- It's a requirement for entry into several countries, mainly in West Africa, regardless of your point of departure (see table below).
- It may be a requirement to enter certain countries if you have recently traveled in countries in the "endemic zone" (see map on following page).

Yellow Fever in Africa

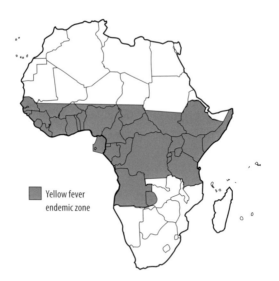

Yellow fever
endemic zone

Yellow Fever in South America

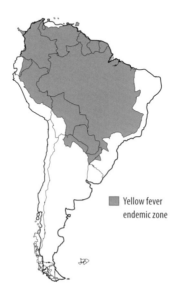

Yellow fever
endemic zone

- It would be recommended, that is, probably not a bad idea, to be vaccinated if you are traveling to a country where there is a current outbreak of YF or where there is potential transmission of the virus.

Some examples:

- To enter Rwanda or Ghana or French Guiana, a YF shot is required, no matter where you came from.
- To enter Brazil after passing through Bolivia (in the YF zone), or to enter Egypt or South Africa after spending time in Tanzania (in the YF zone), would require a YF shot.
- To trek in the jungles of Peru, it would be recommended to get vaccinated against YF, though it is not a requirement.

Countries that require yellow fever vaccination for entry from North America	
Benin	Ivory Coast
Burkino Faso	Liberia
Cameroon	Mali
Central African Republic	Mauritania
Congo	Niger
French Guiana	Rwanda
Gabon	São Tomé and Principé
Ghana	Togo

YF vaccine consists of one dose which is valid and protective for ten years. It needs to be given at least ten days before entering the country. As it is a "live" vaccine, it should not be given to pregnant women or immunosuppressed travelers. Nor should it be given to those allergic to eggs. Travelers

19

Pre-Travel Inoculation

who cannot receive the vaccine, but who insist on traveling to YF countries should receive a "Certificate of Medical Contraindication," or perhaps consider altering their itinerary. YF vaccine can be given to children as young as six months, but preferably not until nine months. Side effects are usually mild and may not appear until 5 to 10 days after vaccination.

However, a severe but rare reaction, known as yellow fever vaccine-associated viscerotropic disease (YEL-AVD) has been reported in the past decade, and several cases have proven fatal. The reaction, which resembles an actual case of YF, has occurred mainly in those over 60. Therefore, if you are over 60 and require the vaccine solely for "bureaucratic" reasons (e.g., traveling from the Andes in Peru where there is no actual risk into Brazil), you might request a certificate of contraindication. If you will potentially be exposed to YF though, the vaccine is recommended. Discuss this with your travel health professional.

Meningococcal disease — Vaccination against the four preventable strains of this bacterium (A, C, Y, W-135) is a requirement for religious pilgrims going to Mecca in Saudi Arabia to observe Hajj or Umrah. Up to three million people from all corners of the earth crowd together for Hajj, so this requirement is not unreasonable. Read below for more information.

RECOMMENDED VACCINATIONS

Hepatitis A — This is a viral infection of the liver which is transmitted through infected food or water or from person to person. While it is not uncommon in North America, the risk of contracting it is much greater in less developed countries, due to a relative lack of hygiene and sanitation (i.e., poverty). After an incubation period of between 14 and 45 days, you may become ill with fever, nausea, abdominal pain, loss of appetite, weakness and fatigue. This is followed by a darkening of the urine and jaundice (a yellowing of the skin and the whites of the eyes).

There is no specific treatment for hepatitis A, and thankfully it usually resolves on its own, though some may have a prolonged recovery. There is no "carrier state," nor are there long-term complications as can occur with hepatitis B and C. In children under the age of 6, the majority of cases, though not all, are asymptomatic, but these kids may return home and infect other susceptible people. In adults over 50, the mortality rate may be as high as 2 percent; not a benign disease.

Vaccination against hepatitis A is recommended for all travelers off to areas of higher risk. Practically speaking, this means almost anywhere outside of North America, Western Europe, Australia, New Zealand and Japan. Five stars and up is always safer than no stars or fewer, but remember, you are only as safe as the last person who handled your food.

Many people who grew up in less developed countries or those who can recall having "yellow jaundice" are probably immune to hepatitis A. This can be checked with a simple blood test.

There are three commercially available vaccines against hepatitis A (Avaxim®, Havrix® and Vaqta®). They are all equally effective and are interchangeable. They will provide protection even if given at the last minute on the way to the airport. One dose of the vaccine provides protection for at least a year. After that, a booster or second dose should give lifelong protection. Hepatitis A vaccine is also available in combination with hepatitis B vaccine (Twinrix®) or with a typhoid vaccine (Vivaxim® or Hepatyrix®).

Hepatitis B — This is another viral infection of the liver, which is transmitted through blood, blood products and unprotected sex. A pregnant mother who is a carrier may pass it on to her

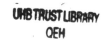

baby. It differs from hepatitis A in that it is much more likely to cause severe illness initially (fulminant hepatitis). About 5 percent of those who are infected go on to become chronic carriers of the virus, which may lead to chronic hepatitis, cirrhosis and liver cancer. This happens more often in kids.

In North America, about 3 percent of our population may carry the hepatitis B virus. In parts of Asia and Africa, this figure may be as high as 15 percent. So, travelers off to these areas are at higher risk, particularly if they are away for longer times, engage in casual sex or do not have access to "good" medical care. While higher-risk travelers definitely need to be protected against hepatitis B, one could make the sensible case that all travelers should be immunized. Once done, it will protect you for life no matter where or how you travel.

Children in most western countries receive hepatitis B vaccine routinely, but the ages at which they receive it may differ. As well, many people who grew up in endemic countries may be immune, and a blood test will prove immunity. There are two available vaccines, Engerix B® and Recombivax®. There are a few different schedules for these vaccines, depending upon the brand, the age and the amount of time you have. While the traditional schedule takes 6 months, it may be accelerated to as little as 21 days. Two doses of the vaccine, while not as effective as three, are still worthwhile if that is all that time allows.

This vaccine should provide lifelong protection, and blood tests to measure immunity are not recommended unless you are at particularly high risk. When combined with Havrix® (hepatitis A vaccine), we get Twinrix®, which provides dual protection for life. This can be given according to the same schedules as hepatitis B vaccine.

There are no vaccines available against hepatitis C (or HIV), whose transmission is the same as hepatitis B, or hepatitis E, a food- and water-borne viral infection which is particularly serious in pregnant women.

Typhoid fever — Typhoid fever is caused by the bacterium *Salmonella typhi*, and is transmitted via infected food and water. It can involve the bloodstream, the lungs, liver, spleen, intestine and brain. Symptoms include fever, headache, cough, confusion, abdominal pain and sometimes intestinal bleeding and a rash. While transmitted in the same way as diarrhea and hepatitis A, it is much less common. It's treatable with antibiotics such as ciprofloxacin, but antibiotic resistance is becoming an ever-increasing problem.

While the infection can be contracted wherever there is poor hygiene and sanitation, it is most commonly imported from countries such as India, Pakistan, Bangladesh, Haiti, the Philippines and Mexico (probably because of the huge number of people who travel there). My point is that not everyone who deserves a hepatitis A shot also needs typhoid vaccine. It should be reserved for the higher-risk travelers, especially the VFRs (see Special Travelers). Paratyphoid fever is a similar, though usually milder, infection passed in the same way as typhoid. There is no longer a vaccine against it, so food and water precautions are again essential.

There is an oral vaccine against typhoid (Vivotif®) and two similar injectable vaccines (Typhim Vi® and Typherix®). The former provides protection for about five years, and the latter, for two to three years. Vivotif® is a "live" vaccine and should not be given to pregnant women or the immunosuppressed. Both vaccines provide about 60 to 70 percent protection. Many people are diagnosed with typhoid fever in Africa and elsewhere. This is probably not because of their poor eating habits or imperfect vaccines, but rather because the infection is overdiagnosed.

Combined vaccines against both hepatitis A and typhoid fever, Vivaxim® or Hepatyrix®, are a convenient idea for those warranting both vaccines.

Meningococcal disease — Meningococcal disease is caused by the bacterium *Neisseria meningitidis*, which is transmitted from person to person via close contact such as coughing, sneezing or direct contact (kissing, sharing coffee cups, etc.). It may involve the blood (meningococcemia) or the brain and spinal cord (meningitis). The symptoms may include fever, headache, vomiting, irritability, changes in the level of consciousness and a stiff neck. It's usually accompanied by a petechial (small bruises) rash. While it often begins like a mild illness, it may quickly progress to shock, convulsions, coma and death within 24 to 48 hours of the onset. Even with optimal therapy, the mortality rate may range from 5 to 15 percent, and survivors may be left with significant disability.

There are five strains of this bacterium, four of which can be prevented by vaccination (A, C, Y, W-135). There is not yet a vaccine against group B. This quadrivalent vaccine will likely become a routine vaccine for children (and will replace the previous one that protected only against group C). It can also be administered to those who have previously received the vaccine against group C. The newer vaccine (Menactra®) not only prevents disease, but also prevents people from becoming asymptomatic carriers of the infection.

For travelers, the vaccine is recommended for those spending a few weeks or more in the meningitis belt of Africa (see map), or to areas where there have been recent outbreaks of meningitis. If there will be lots of contact with local people, it is that much more important. In Africa, transmission is greatest during the windy dry season, which extends from December through May. The risk is greatest in young children. As mentioned above, the vaccine is a requirement for religious pilgrims visiting Saudi Arabia. Children here are now routinely inoculated against meningococcal disease; hence, you see it here in all the sections — Routine, Required and Recommended.

Meningococcal Meningitis in Africa

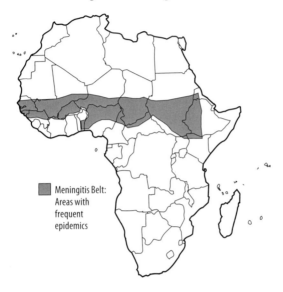

Meningitis Belt:
Areas with
frequent
epidemics

Japanese encephalitis (JE) — JE is a viral infection of the brain that occurs in rural parts of Asia and Southeast Asia (see map on following page). It is transmitted by the Culex mosquito, which bites between dusk and dawn, particularly in areas with rice paddies and pig farming. The infection is seasonal in temperate climates, being more prevalent between May and October. In more tropical areas, it may be year-round and associated with monsoon rainfalls.

The vast majority of those who become infected do not become ill. In those who do, it begins with a flu-like illness with fever, chills, headache, nausea and vomiting. Confusion, agitation, seizures and Parkinsonian-like movement disorders may develop. Of those who survive serious illness, many are left with significant disability. I believe the soldier in the book *The Cider House Rules* returned with JE. Thankfully, JE is quite rare in travelers. Children and the elderly are at greatest risk.

Japanese Encephalitis

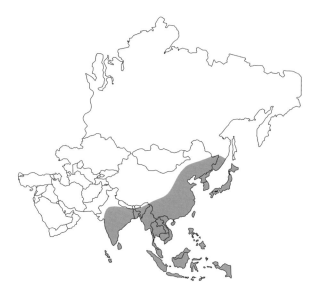

A new vaccine against JE, Ixiaro® (who makes up these names?), has recently become available. It consists of two doses given a month apart, and it provides more than 90 percent protection. It has fewer side effects than the previously available vaccine but is not recommended in pregnancy or those under the age of 18. Other effective vaccines (e.g., JE-Vax®) may be available locally and for less money in country. Ixiaro® is recommended for higher-risk travelers spending a month or more in areas of risk during the transmission season. So the person hopscotching from Bangkok to Chang Mai to Kuala Lumpur to Angkor Wat to Hanoi to Hong Kong in two weeks probably does not warrant this vaccine.

Rabies — Thank God I have never had a patient/traveler/volunteer with rabies, as the infection, once you become ill, is 100 percent fatal. But I have had no shortage of frantic calls from travelers and their mothers about dog (and monkey) bites. There are other animals that can transmit rabies (cats, skunks, racoons, bats, foxes), but if you can concentrate on dogs I will be happy.

Rabies is a viral infection of the central nervous system (the brain) transmitted by the saliva from infected dogs and other less important furry animals. This usually means a bite that has broken the skin, but could also include a lick over a break in the skin. Recently, it was discovered that eating infected dog meat, even if it is cooked, can lead to rabies.

There is not much point in describing the symptoms of rabies, because if you have them you will probably die. Some of you are old enough to have seen the movie *Old Yeller*, where the beloved dog was irritable and foaming at the mouth! In fact, you cannot, I repeat, cannot, tell the difference between a rabid dog and a non-rabid one. Over here, we may have the luxury of looking at the dog's collar, speaking to the owner, or quarantining the animal at the local vet. One rarely has that luxury in the middle of India or Thailand or Togo! A bite must be assumed to be a potentially rabid one.

One can be vaccinated against rabies before departure. This requires three doses of vaccine, on days 0 – 7 – 21 or 28. There are several safe vaccines (Imovax®, Rabipur®, Rabavert®, Verorab®, Rabivac®), and they are interchangeable if necessary. Rabies vaccine is very expensive (in North America). When I wrote my first book, it cost about $100 per dose. That is more than $200 per dose now. Therefore, it is a vaccine we reserve for the higher-risk traveler. Children are at higher risk because they are more likely to play with dogs and not report a bite. As well, a bite in a child will likely be closer to the brain. Spelunkers (they explore caves) or vets would also be at higher risk.

Rabies vaccine can also be given intradermally (.1 cc just under the skin-like a TB test) in one-tenth the dose. If you are traveling as a family or with others, this may be one way to reduce the cost.

If you have received pre-exposure vaccination and you get bitten, immediately wash the wound thoroughly for 15 minutes with soap and water and disinfect with alcohol or iodine if available. Then you still need two doses of one of the above rabies vaccines ASAP on days 0 and 3. Do this, and you will be fine!

If you have not received pre-exposure vaccination, wash the wound, and then you need a dose of human rabies immune globulin (HRIG), also ASAP (it is never too late to begin). This should ideally be injected into the site of the wound. If that is not possible, some or all of it may be given into the buttock. This provides some immediate antibodies and protection. This must be followed by five doses (recently changed to four by CDC) on days 0 – 3 – 7 – 14 and 28.

HRIG is not always available in every country. If it isn't, you need to travel to somewhere that it is. My experience tells me that not every local doctor will be as concerned about a dog bite as I am. They may not suggest vaccination, or perhaps only with vaccine and not HRIG. They may be right, but I don't take that chance, and neither should you.

The rabies virus travels up the course of the nerve until it reaches the brain. This may take a few days, or months. It may depend upon where you were bitten. But, you always have time to get to the proper treatment, whether it is available locally or requires a flight home.

Rabies vaccine probably lasts for life, but if you are at high risk, you may want to check your antibody level every two years or so.

So my instructions to travelers are as follows:

- Don't play with dogs, monkeys, or other furry animals (puppies are just little dogs).
- If you get bitten, wash the wound thoroughly.
- Go to a big city and ask for the proper rabies vaccine.

- Call me (not everyone should call me) or whoever can help ensure that you get the proper treatment.

Traveler's Diarrhea (Enterotoxigenic *E. coli*) — This bacterium is probably responsible for 50 to 60 percent of the diarrhea in travelers, depending upon the destination. The diarrhea is usually relatively mild, often happening on the third day after arrival, consisting of three loose bowel movements a day, and lasting for three days. Dukoral® is an oral vaccine that will lower your risk of getting *E. coli* by about 60 percent. Considering that it is responsible for about 50 percent of the diarrhea, it therefore provides approximately 30 percent protection. This may not be as good as other vaccines, but remember it is a common infection.

The vaccine consists of two doses, taken a week apart, and should be completed at least a week prior to travel. Its protective effect lasts for about three months. For subsequent trips, if they are within five years, only a single booster dose is necessary. The vaccine tastes OK and is unlikely to have any side effects. Children as young as two can take it, though it is best avoided in pregnant women. This vaccine is appropriate for almost anyone who wants to take it (realizing its limitations), and more so, for higher-risk travelers, such as those with inflammatory bowel disease or young children going to India.

Cholera — This is a bacterial infection (*Vibrio cholera*) of the intestine transmitted via contaminated water, which unfortunately continues to cause severe outbreaks around the world. While some people develop only a mild illness, others may suffer severe watery diarrhea and vomiting, which may quickly progress to dehydration and death if not properly treated. Oral rehydration with ORS (oral rehydration solutions) was "invented" for this illness, and if this does not suffice, then intravenous fluids are needed. Antibiotics such as Cipro® are useful in treating severe cases. This is a disease of extreme poverty. As I write this, the most recent outbreak has been in Zimbabwe. It is highly unlikely to occur in the average, or even the not so average, traveler.

Having said that, Dukoral®, which is used to prevent garden variety Traveler's Diarrhea, was originally intended as a cholera vaccine. In fact, it is more effective against cholera, about 60 percent, and that protection lasts for up to six months. So, for that extremely high-risk traveler, say someone off to a disaster zone or an area with a known cholera outbreak, consider this vaccine.

Tick-borne encephalitis — This is a tick-borne infection of the brain found in rural areas of Eastern and Western Europe. While humans aren't their first choice, ticks are happy to jump off plants, grass and bushes onto unsuspecting hikers, especially during the spring and summer months. It may begin with a flu-like illness, which may be followed by more severe symptoms such as neck stiffness, dizziness, tremors, drowsiness, delirium and coma. It is rarely fatal, but permanent neurological damage may occur.

The vaccine (FSME-Immun®) consists of two doses a month apart, with a booster dose in a year, and then every three years if exposure continues.

Tuberculosis (TB) — TB is a bacterial infection which primarily affects the lungs, though it may also involve the kidney, spinal cord, bowel, bones or lymph nodes. Two million people die each year from TB, mainly in poorer countries. One third of the world's population is infected (not necessarily ill), and 5 to 10 percent of those will become sick and infectious at some point in their lives. Those with HIV/AIDS are at the highest risk.

TB is transmitted via respiratory droplets, that is, coughing and sneezing. It usually requires prolonged contact with infectious individuals under crowded conditions, as is seen with extreme poverty. It is a treatable infection, but treatment requires multiple drugs for many months, and drug resistance and poor compliance make it a very difficult infection to treat.

Infection with TB is a fairly small risk to most travelers, but it may occur. Those who are at the greatest risk are travelers going off to highly endemic areas for longer periods of time, and who will have lots of exposure to the local population. Long-term volunteers, VFRs and missionaries fit this description. Becoming infected, or having "latent" TB, does not mean you are sick or contagious, but there is a risk of this happening in the future, particularly if you become immunosuppressed.

There is a fair bit of controversy regarding immunization to prevent TB. Most of the world outside of North America routinely administers BCG to children at birth. This is supposed to prevent TB. In fact, from the studies that have been done, it is not absolutely certain whether BCG works best in certain age groups, against certain forms of TB, and in certain geographic areas.

The North American approach has always been to do a TB skin test (Mantoux test) prior to travel. This test is usually normal or negative, unless there has been past exposure or vaccination with BCG. Being negative, the usual plan is to repeat the test one to two months after return. In this way, we detect those who have "converted" from negative to positive. It is this group who is at higher risk of developing active TB, and hence would benefit from a course of medication, usually INH (isoniazid), as chemoprophylaxis for six to twelve months. Pre-travel TB skin testing need not be done in every traveler; rather, it should be reserved for those with longer (more than three months), higher-risk travel plans.

What are the side effects of vaccines?

For the most part, the side effects are mild, consisting of localized soreness and tenderness at the site of injection within the first 48 hours. Flu-like symptoms such as a fever and muscle aches occur, but are less common. Allergic reactions tend to be quite rare, but they can happen. Serious reactions can occur, as in the case of yellow fever, but they are also rare. The risks and benefits of inoculation should be discussed with your doctor.

What is not so rare is vasovagal syncope, or a simple fainting spell. The combination of anticipation, multiple injections and a bit of pain is sometimes enough to provoke this reaction. An empty stomach and three layers of clothing don't help either. Teens seem to do most of the fainting. Previous fainters should alert the doctor or nurse so that they can lie down after the injection.

If you are acutely ill or feverish, you and your doctor should probably postpone your vaccinations. Runny noses, sprained ankles, tension headaches and tummy aches probably don't qualify as "sick," and it would be safe to proceed in such situations. There is no shortage of people out there extolling the dangers of vaccination. If you choose to believe everything that you hear, I suggest you do so at your own risk.

A few more points about vaccines

- While some vaccines can be given at the last minute, others can't or may require a series of shots (e.g., rabies, hepatitis B and JE). So if possible, give yourself several weeks to get your vaccines before traveling.
- Make sure you receive a written record of your shots.
- You may receive several vaccines at the same sitting. You will just be a little bit sorer in more places.

- If you are a known "fainter," let the doctor or nurse know in advance. If you feel like you are going to faint, lie down and elevate your legs.
- Remain in the waiting room for 20 minutes after your injection(s) because allergic reactions (and delayed fainting spells) may occur.
- Some vaccines are given as a series. If you failed to complete the series, it is probably not necessary to start again at the beginning. Continue where you left off.
- The recommended interval between shots in a series, such as hepatitis A or even rabies, may be lengthened if necessary, but not shortened.
- Vaccines are very effective (this may vary a bit) and safe in my opinion. But they are not an excuse to ignore personal protective measures, such as insect repellents, food and water precautions, practicing safe sex and avoiding dogs.

So roll up your sleeve(s). Get your shots, and enjoy your trip.

Summary of Pre-travel Vaccinations

Disease	Vaccine	Course	Duration
hepatitis A	Avaxim® (SP)* Havrix® (GSK) Vaqta® (Merck)*	single dose good for 1 year; booster at 6–12 months	life
hepatitis B	Engerix B® (GSK)* Recombivax® (Merck)	0–1–6 months; accelerated: 0–1–2–12 months; 0–7–21, 0–14–28 days, booster at 12 months	life
hepatitis A / B	Twinrix® (GSK)*	0–1–6 months; may also be accelerated as above if necessary	life
typhoid fever	Typhim-Vi® (SP)* Typherix® (GSK)* Vivotif® (Berna)	single dose oral: 4 doses on alternate days	2 years (U.S.) 3 years (Canada) 5 yrs
yellow fever	YF-Vax® (SP)*	single dose	10 yrs
meningococcal disease	Menactra® (SP)* (A,C,Y,W-135)	single dose	likely 5 years or more
rabies	Imovax® (HDCV)(SP)* RabAvert® (PCEC) (Chiron)	pre-exposure: 0–7–21 (or 28) days post-exposure: 0–3 days if previously vaccinated; 0–3–7–14–28 if not, and must receive human rabies immune globulin (HRIG)	check immunity every 2 years if exposure continues
Japanese encephalitis	Ixiaro® (Novartis)*	0 and 28 days	likely 2 years or more
tick-borne encephalitis	FSME-Immun® (Baxter)	2 doses, 1–3 months apart	booster at 12 months, and then every 3 years
cholera	Dukoral®	0 and 7 days	6 months
E. coli (TD)	Dukoral®	0 and 7 days	3 months

*GSK = Glaxo SmithKline
*SP = Sanofi Pasteur
Note: Check dosages and instructions with doctor or pharmacist.

34

ARE YOU FIT TO FLY?

Most aircrafts cruise at about 30,000 feet. Pressurization of the plane makes this equivalent to about 8,000 feet above sea level, or the altitude of Aspen, Colorado. Most people have no problem with this, considering we are mainly sitting like couch potatoes during the flight. But for some, this and other aspects of flight might present a problem.

- **Anemia** — The usual adult hemoglobin (red blood cell count) is between 12 and 15 (120 to 150 in Canada). Anyone whose hemoglobin is less than 8.5 (85 in Canada) may have difficulty during flight due to the decreased level of oxygen. Supplemental oxygen can be arranged in advance, or travel can be postponed. People with sickle cell anemia, an inherited disorder in black people, may also be at risk.

- **Pregnancy** — Women are not permitted on international flights after 36 weeks of gestation because of the risk of early delivery. (I am comfortable with fainters, but not childbirth!)

- **Scuba diving** — Divers are at risk of decompression illness if they fly in a low-pressure environment too soon after diving. The accepted safe interval between the last dive (depending upon the depth) and flight is 12–24 hours.

- **Heart and lung disease** — People with severe cardio-vascular disease, such as unstable angina, congestive heart failure or a recent heart attack or stroke, should preferably not fly. The same goes for those with severe COPD (Chronic Obstructive Pulmonary Disease), acute asthma or a chest infection.

- **Psychiatric** — Those with an unstable condition such as psychosis should not fly unless they are accompanied by a psychiatrist or psychiatric nurse.

SPECIAL TRAVELERS

Every traveler is different. Travelers go to different locations for different reasons and they come in all sizes and sexes. As well, they may have different medical problems or conditions.

TRAVELERS WITH CHRONIC MEDICAL CONDITIONS

The Boy Scout motto "Be Prepared" applies to all travelers, especially to those with chronic medical problems. There are countless medical conditions that travelers travel with, such as diabetes, heart and lung disease, inflammatory bowel disease and arthritis being the most important conditions I see in my practice.

Why are they different?

- Some may in fact not be fit to travel in the first place.
- They are likely on more medications than others.
- They may be more likely to become ill while away and require medical care.
- They may be adversely affected by the conditions of their destination, such as the altitude, pollution, climate and local food.
- Infections such as Traveler's Diarrhea may impact them more than others.

How can you minimize the risks?

Of course this might depend upon your particular medical problem, but I think that some advice applies to everyone.

- Give yourself plenty of time to prepare for your trip, not just to get the recommended inoculations, but to ensure that you are in as good shape as possible before you leave. This would involve a trip to your doctor!

- Carry a more than adequate supply of your medications and supplies (e.g., lancets for blood glucose monitoring), and preferably keep them in your hand luggage. Carry an up-to-date list of your pills as well.
- Take a list of your personal physician, specialists, etc., with their contact numbers.
- Carry a summary of your medical history and perhaps copies of a recent electrocardiogram or blood tests if applicable.
- Wear a Medic Alert® bracelet if you have allergies, bionic parts, are on blood thinners, have a pacemaker or other significant issues.
- Contact the airline in advance if you will need special seating, supplemental oxygen, boarding assistance, a special diet or anything else.
- Ensure that you have adequate medical and travel insurance.
- Should you have other physical disabilities such as arthritis or depend upon a wheelchair, make sure that your transportation and accommodation are accessible in advance.
- Plan your trip sensibly. Be aware of your limitations if you have any. Having said that, Chris Waddell, a paraplegic, just conquered Kilimanjaro on a custom-made four-wheel mountain bike! Limitations are relative!

For those with **heart disease**:

- Avoid traveling if you have unstable angina, symptomatic congestive heart failure or serious irregularities of your heart rhythm.
- Delay travel for at least three weeks following a heart attack or coronary bypass surgery. Air travel may be undertaken within a few days of having an angioplasty or stent inserted.

For those with **diabetes**:

- Get a doctor's note if you are carrying syringes or lancets.
- It is likely that your diet and activity will change while you are away, so the dosages of your insulin or oral medications might need to be adjusted. Therefore, close glucose monitoring is essential during travel.
- When crossing many time zones by plane, it is not critical that you have perfect control of your blood sugar. Rather, your goal should be to avoid becoming hypoglycemic (low blood sugar) or too hyperglycemic (high blood sugar).
- Always carry a quick source of sugar — sweet candies, granola bars, orange juice — in case your sugar does dip too low.

For those with **inflammatory bowel disease (IBD)**:

- Be exceedingly careful with your food and water.
- Consider taking the vaccine, Dukoral®, prior to travel to reduce your risk of getting diarrhea.
- Should you get sick remember that most cases of diarrhea in travelers are caused by bacteria, so the prompt use of an antibiotic such as Cipro®, Zithromax® or Xifaxan® for one to three days might give you the quickest relief. Prophylactic or preventative antibiotics are also an option for the short-term traveler with IBD.

For those with **chronic lung diseases**:

- Make sure that you are immunized against pneumonia and the appropriate flu strains.
- Consider wearing an N95 mask in crowds.
- Carry antibiotics to use in case you think you have a respiratory infection.

- Avoid the most polluted destinations such as Kathmandu, Manila, Mumbai and Mexico City.
- Request supplemental oxygen for your flight in advance if your doctor feels it is necessary.

TRAVELERS WITH IMMUNE SYSTEM DISORDERS

Our immune system is one of the many things in life we take for granted. That is, until we no longer have a properly functioning one. This can come about for many reasons, but is usually the result of certain conditions or infections (e.g., leukemia, HIV/AIDS and removal of the spleen) or the medications used to treat these and other conditions (e.g., chemotherapy, steroids and immune modulators). Many "autoimmune" diseases such as lupus erythematosus, inflammatory bowel disease and multiple sclerosis probably do not result in immunosuppression on their own, but their treatments often do.

An ever increasing number of travelers are immunosuppressed and require special consideration, preferably from a travel medicine specialist and/or their appropriate specialist.

Why are they different?

- They may be more susceptible to various infections while traveling. Some of these would be considered unusual or opportunistic infections (e.g., pneumocystis pneumonia and cryptosporidiosis). Others are available to everyone but may be more severe in someone who is immunosuppressed, such as malaria or diarrheal disease (*Salmonella* and *Campylobacter* infections).
- Live vaccines (e.g., yellow fever, oral typhoid and oral polio) are not recommended for these travelers. This may preclude visiting certain destinations.
- While most of the vaccines are "killed" or

"inactivated" and considered safe, they may not produce the desired immune response and protection in the immuno suppressed.

- Certain countries may require a negative HIV test as a condition of entry. This would more likely apply to longer-stay travelers on a work permit.

Patients infected with HIV can assess their immune status by having their CD4 count checked. Anything under 200 is considered immunosuppressed. A count of between 200 and 500 may mean some extent of immunosuppression. In the case of oral steroids, a daily dose of 10 mg per day for more than two weeks would be significant. Steroid inhalers, creams and injections do not increase risk. Immune modulators, such as Humira®, Enbrel® and Remicade® are used for a number of conditions such as Crohn's disease, rheumatoid arthritis and psoriasis, and they do have the potential to lower immunity.

How can you minimize the risks?

- See a travel medicine specialist who can advise you regarding the safety, or lack thereof, of certain vaccines (mainly yellow fever, oral typhoid and oral polio).
- Delay travel to certain areas until your immunity has improved with time or treatment.
- Killed or inactivated vaccines are safe and you should receive the recommended ones.
- If you must travel to a country where yellow fever is a risk, you might want a Certificate of Medical Contraindication. You may also have to weigh the risk of the vaccine against the risk of disease. Perhaps visiting Machu Picchu in Peru but not the Amazon or other yellow fever areas would be the best idea.
- Travelers who have been on chemotherapy should

delay receiving live vaccines for three months after chemotherapy has been completed.

- If your spleen has been removed, or you have sickle cell anemia, you should be immunized against *Haemophilus influenza*, pneumococcal and meningococcal disease.
- Pay particular attention to food and water precautions and insect avoidance.
- Consider using a prophylactic antibiotic such as ciprofloxacin (Cipro®) or rifaximin (Xifaxan®) for the short term prevention of Traveler's Diarrhea.
- In the case of hepatitis B vaccine, a higher dose may be used to achieve good immunity.
- Take along your pertinent medical records in case you need medical care abroad, and know where you will get your medical care before you need it.
- Ensure that your medical insurance covers your preexisting conditions.

PREGNANT TRAVELERS

There's a time and place for everything, and when it comes to travel, women must sometimes decide whether pregnancy is the time and Tibet the place. Certainly, pregnancy should not be a bar to traveling, but it is necessary to consider some of the additional risks involved and to take measures to reduce these risks.

Why are they different?

- Especially in the first three months, they may feel extremely tired or nauseated.
- They may experience complications of pregnancy, such as bleeding and miscarriage in the first trimester, and premature labor at almost any time.
- The choice of medications to treat diarrheal disease and prevent malaria is limited.

- Malaria is a much greater threat to mom and her baby than to other travelers.
- Live vaccines, such as for yellow fever, are contraindicated.
- They are "hypercoagulable," (more prone to developing blood clots on long flights or drives).
- Certain activities, such as mountain climbing and scuba diving, can adversely affect both mom and baby.
- They tend to get a bit "bulky," especially in the last few months, so their mobility may be limited.

How can you minimize the risks?

- Avoid "live" vaccines such as yellow fever, oral typhoid and measles; the "killed" vaccines are safe in pregnancy, though I prefer to administer them after the first trimester if at all possible.
- Chloroquine for the prevention of malaria is safe in pregnancy, but is effective only in a few places — Haiti, Dominican Republic, rural Central America and the Middle East.
- In chloroquine-resistant areas (everywhere else), mefloquine (Lariam®) is considered safe in the second and third trimesters, and would be the best choice in the first. DEET is safe in pregnancy.
- Another option would be to postpone your trip until after your pregnancy.
- Follow the "*Boil it, bottle it* ..." mantra religiously. Imodium® should be avoided. If an antibiotic is used, it should be Zithromax® (azithromycin).
- On a long haul flight, drink plenty of fluids, get up and move around and consider wearing compression stockings.
- Don't plan extended periods of time above 12,000

feet. In addition to altitude sickness, you may not be near adequate medical care.

- Scuba diving is not recommended. Snorkel!
- Don't fly after 36 weeks of pregnancy. The airline won't take you! Check out your medical insurance if you plan to fly earlier.
- The best time to travel is in your second trimester.

FEMALE TRAVELERS

While most of what I have discussed in this book applies equally to men and women, there are a few issues that are mainly or exclusively applicable to women.

Why are they different?

- If of the right age, they may become pregnant.
- They need to be responsible for their own birth control and STI prevention.
- Many will get their menstrual periods while away and will need feminine hygiene products.
- They may be subjected to sexual harassment or unacceptable treatment that would not happen back home.
- They may be more susceptible to the side effects of antimalarials such as doxycycline and mefloquine.
- They tend to have more common sense and exhibit less risk-taking behavior compared to men.

How can you minimize the risks?

- Young women are more prone to the side effects of mefloquine (Lariam®). Try starting it a few weeks before you depart to see if it bothers you, or consider other antimalarials such as doxycycline, Malarone® or primaquine.

- If you plan to be sexually active while away, take enough birth control pills to last your entire trip and more. Newer preparations such as Seasonale® have an 84 days on/7 days off schedule. This is quite safe and effective and will help you avoid a "tropical" period if you wish!

- Don't count on male partners to carry condoms. Carry your own, preferably "Western" condoms that have not sat in your oven-like glove compartment for three months!

- Female condoms boast a high degree of efficacy when it comes to preventing pregnancy (though not as high as the birth control pill) and sexually trans-mitted infections — that is, if used properly and every time. The female condom, which is made from polyurethane, can be inserted into the vagina up to eight hours before intercourse. It may be used with both water-based and oil-based lubricants.

- Depo-Provera® is an injectable form of birth control which must be given every 12 weeks. It's more than 99 percent effective in preventing pregnancy, and it's available worldwide. Side effects may include irregu-lar bleeding, increased appetite, headaches, depres-sion, abdominal pain and increased or decreased sex drive. These unwanted effects are not reversed until the medication wears off (up to 12 weeks), but do tend to get better with time.

- Menstrual periods often go AWOL during travel. This is OK as long as you know you are not pregnant.

- Some women may choose to carry "the morning after pill" for emergency contraception. These may consist of combination estrogen/progestin (e.g., Ovral®), progestin alone (e.g., Plan B®), or Mifepristone. Availability will vary around the world. While they are all at least 90 percent effective in preventing pregnancy, they should not be counted on as a form of birth control. They must be taken up to five days after having sex, but the sooner the better.

- Vaginal infections may happen at the best of times, and traveling, especially in warm climates, may make the problem worse. Antibiotics, including the antimalarial doxycycline, can also contribute to this problem. Take along a vaginal cream such as Monistat® or a single-dose tablet like Diflucan® in case you do develop a yeast infection.

- Be aware of the need for PEP (post exposure prophylaxis – See Chapter 3) if you are sexually assaulted.

- Take along plenty of your favorite feminine hygiene products, as they may be expensive or not available at your destination. One solution recommended to me by a worldly female traveler is "The Keeper" (www.keeper.com), a small, bell-shaped natural gum rubber menstrual cap that is worn internally. It is a comfortable, hygienic, sanitary, safe alternative to tampons and pads. It's very easy to use (so I am told), and one cap will last for many years, according to the manufacturer.

- Pay attention to your personal safety. Maybe wear a cheap wedding band, and have some stories ready to tell about your "husband and children." Don't accept a drink unless you have seen it poured. Dress with common sense and respect for the local culture. Whenever possible, do not walk or travel alone. If there are "women only" buses or train cars, take them. They are there for a reason.

45

CHILDREN

Some would argue that if children are too young to remember a trip years down the road, then leave them at home. But with a bit of extra planning and patience, it can be a wonderful experience.

Why are they different?

- Their endurance, desires and culinary preferences will be different than yours.
- In the case of visiting friends and relatives, they are often high risk travelers.
- They may be too young for certain vaccinations.
- They tend to get sick more often, more quickly and sicker than adults.
- Kids are more prone to motion sickness. (See Chapter 2.)

How can you minimize the risks and your stress?

- Plan ahead. Take any supplies like a car seat, diapers and baby foods.
- Take along plenty of things to keep the kids happy: books, dolls, games, etc.
- Ensure that the children's identification papers are in order. If you are traveling as a single parent, a legal document signed by the non-traveling parent should be obtained.
- Learn how to recognize and treat common medical conditions in your children, and carry adequate medications.
- Consider MMR (measles-mumps-rubella) vaccine for children between 6 and 12 months of age if you will be taking the baby to a lesser-developed country.

- If you will be spending a longer time in Africa, India or Southeast Asia, consider pre-exposure vaccination against rabies for your children. Teach them to stay away from dogs!
- Try the Emla® patch to minimize the pain of the injections.
- Keep your kids from getting insect bites. (See Chapter 4.)
- With respect to antimalarials, mefloquine (Lariam®) is usually well tolerated in kids as long as it is taken with lots of food and water. Malarone® may cause mouth ulcers, especially in children with braces! Doxycycline is not recommended under the age of 8.
- Kids get sicker with Traveler's Diarrhea. The choice of antibiotic for more serious diarrhea in those 16 and under is Zithromax® (azithromycin). (See Chapter 2.)
- Make sure the environment where you are living is safe. Take a night light for small children, and outlet covers to use in hotel rooms. And don't forget the sunscreen!

BUSINESS TRAVELERS

Many people envy the business traveler — first class flights (not always), luxurious hotels (if you're lucky), expense accounts, frequent flyer points and a chance to get out of the office! But there is the other side to it — rush to the airport, endless lines at check-in, flight delays, work seven days a week, miss your children's hockey/soccer/karate tournament, jet lag and piles of work on your return!

Why are they different?
- It is often short term, one to two weeks of travel.
- They usually travel alone.

- They are traveling at someone else's expense.
- They are often repeat travelers.
- They work hard while they are away.
- The impact of any illness, such as Traveler's Diarrhea, may be greater on a short business trip than it would be on your year-long volunteer stint.
- They usually miss their families very much.

It is the employer's responsibility to provide their employee with a safe workplace. Back home, that might include a safety helmet, steel-toed boots or earplugs. In far off countries, it is protective immunization, antimalarials, safe transportation and much more.

How can you minimize the risks?

- Get immunized according to your destination and other risk factors; consider Twinrix® (hepatitis A and B) which will last the rest of your life.
- Dukoral® will provide you with moderate protection against Traveler's Diarrhea. Prophylactic antibiotics can also be considered for the "I can't afford to get sick" business traveler.
- Don't even think about unprotected sex while you are away. Use condoms if you are sexually active abroad!
- Malarone® is a great choice for malaria prevention in short-term travelers.
- Consider getting some advice or medication to deal with jet lag. (See Chapter 2.)
- Try to reduce your stress level — fly first class if you can! Keep in touch with your family by phone or e-mail. Get some fresh air and exercise at your destination.
- Practise meditation, yoga, or take your iPod.
- Carry a small first aid kit and sewing kit to look after minor ailments and repairs.

VISITING FRIENDS AND RELATIVES

VFRs are those who are traveling abroad in order to visit friends and relatives. The acronym was introduced a few years ago by Dr. Jay Keystone. It is not meant to denote those who drive from Toronto to Cleveland to see their college classmates, nor those who fly to Orlando for a family reunion. Rather, I am thinking about the Indian family visiting their parents and grandparents in the Punjab, or the Ghanaian-born family taking their kids home for the first time to see their roots and relatives. Studies and experience have shown us that VFRs are higher risk travelers — they become ill more often, especially with infections such as diarrhea, malaria and typhoid fever.

Why are they different?

If I can be permitted to generalize (as usual):

- They generally travel to poorer, less developed countries, such as Ghana, Nigeria, Ethiopia, India, Pakistan and the Philippines (among many others).
- They are often traveling for longer periods of time.
- They are more likely to be visiting smaller towns in rural areas, with less access to good hygiene, sanitation and medical care.
- They will have more contact with the local population.
- The adults often feel a sense of immunity or protection from disease because they grew up there. This may be true in the case of hepatitis A or B, but not for most of the infections that await them, especially malaria.
- They more often travel with their children, who are often numerous and quite young.
- They will likely be repeat travelers.

- English may be their second language and they may have difficulty understanding all of the travel health information.
- They may not be able to afford the costs of vaccinations and antimalarials.

How can you minimize the risks?

Providing pre-travel counseling to VFRs can be challenging for all of the above reasons. Because of their higher risk, it is critical that parents understand the seriousness of some of the infections to which they and their children will be exposed. Sometimes it is the older children who must explain things to their parents. The rules, vaccinations, pills and treatments are no different in VFRs than in any other traveler, but they might take more explaining and reinforcement. Multilingual office staff in travel clinics, plus handouts in various languages would be beneficial.

MEDICAL CARE ABROAD

Traveling usually conjures up visions of pristine beaches, historic sites and romantic dinners, but sometimes things like appendicitis, kidney stones, diarrhea, dengue fever and hospital fees intervene. So travel prepared and insured.

GETTING PREPARED

If you have significant preexisting medical problems, carry a list of them, along with any pertinent reports on a card or your BlackBerry if you have one. While you're at it, record the names and phone numbers of your doctors in case you need to contact them.

A MedicAlert® bracelet is an effective way of informing the local doctor that you have, for example, diabetes, dangerous allergies, epilepsy, a pacemaker, artificial heart valves or joints, or you are taking blood thinners.

YOUR MEDICATIONS

To avoid medication disasters, pay attention to the following:

- Learn the names of your medications, as just knowing the color and shape of your pills might not be good enough when you lose them. Carry a written list or record them on your BlackBerry. Most drugs go by two names, the generic name and the brand name. The generic name is the actual name of the compound, and the brand name is what the manufacturer likes you to call it. While it's best to know both names, it's imperative that you know at least the generic name, as this will probably be the easiest way to find the equivalent of what you need and least likely to confuse the local doctor.
- Take along more pills then you will need.

- Carry them in their original labeled containers, not in your late mother's pillbox!
- Store your pills in more than one location. The airline may misplace your bags, so carry essential medications also in your carry-on luggage.
- If you are carrying narcotics or syringes and lancets for diabetes, carry an explanatory note from your doctor.

In many countries, especially the less developed ones, most medications are available over the counter, or without a prescription. Often these will be sold in their original packaging, so it's possible — hopefully — to know exactly what you are getting. On the other hand, many doctors and clinics will dispense your pills in flimsy, little plastic bags with labeling that's both illegible and in a foreign language.

What is the quality of medications abroad?

Widespread counterfeiting of medicines, inadequate quality assurance during the manufacturing process and poor storage may all contribute to substandard drugs. It's best to anticipate your medicinal needs before you leave home. When abroad, do your best to shop at the most reputable pharmacy; though sometimes pills will be dispensed by the doctor himself.

INSURANCE

Don't skimp when it comes to your medical and travel insurance.

Medical Insurance — Buy the best that you can afford. The insurance you may have at home, whether it's government sponsored or private, will likely not be adequate should an emergency arise while you are away. Carry proof of your insurance with you at all times. In addition, the cliché "Read the fine print" could never be truer. Your medical insurance should cover you for:

- the costs incurred for all doctors', dentists' and hospital fees
- the costs of any prescribed medications
- medical evacuation to the nearest adequate medical facility, or back home if necessary
- emergency replacement of lost medications or supplies
- emergency cash advances
- assistance in finding medical care abroad

If you have preexisting medical conditions, your insurer will want to know about them. Unfortunately, this may increase the cost of your premium. For those who plan to engage in some higher-risk pursuits, such as climbing Everest, white water rafting, scuba diving or bungee jumping, make sure that injuries resulting from such hazardous activities are covered.

Many doctors and medical facilities abroad may be reluctant to bill your insurance provider directly. Make sure that you have access to the necessary funds should an emergency arise. Retain all receipts for medical services and medications. And don't forget, read the fine print. Some policies may cover only "emergency" medical problems. The definition of "emergency" may be a bit ambiguous.

Travel Insurance — In addition to supplemental medical insurance, you should consider the need for travel insurance. Important features of this plan would be:

- trip cancellation, interruption or delay protection (due to illness involving yourself, your traveling companion or your family, or other factors such as airline strikes, weather and terrorism)

- protection against the default or bankruptcy of suppliers
- replacement of travel documents such as your driver's license or credit cards
- reimbursement for lost luggage or personal possessions
- a 24-hour hotline to provide emergency travel advice and assistance
- legal assistance

Contained in the fine print may be situations that are not covered, such as acts of God (floods, earthquakes, hurricanes, etc.), acts of terrorism or hijacking and wars (declared and undeclared).

How do I locate medical care abroad?

It's always preferable, though not always possible, to know where you will get your medical care before you need it. Here are some ways of accessing medical care while you are away:

- Have your doctor put you in touch with colleagues abroad should you need care.
- Contact your employer or sending agency.
- Call the toll-free number provided by your insurance company.
- Contact your local embassy or consulate for advice.
- Request a visit from the "hotel" doctor.
- Join IAMAT (www.iamat.org), which will provide you with a list of English-speaking doctors abroad.
- Try word of mouth or your guidebook.
- Walk into the first clinic you find!

The quality of medical care around the world varies greatly. In some countries, it may even be faster and more efficient than what you are used to back home. Medical tourists are flocking to India, Thailand and Costa Rica because of their excellent and less-expensive medical facilities. But let me give you some generalizations about "third world" care, which I have gleaned from numerous e-mails and frantic phone calls from abroad:

- Diagnostic facilities are often unreliable or unavailable.
- Doctors often give you more than one diagnosis. In the tropics, the diagnoses of malaria and typhoid are quite popular and often co-exist.
- You may be treated with polypharmacy, that is, multiple different medications to cover more than one diagnosis and several symptoms.
- Local doctors are much more likely to treat you with an injection.

How can I protect myself?

- Try to know where you will go for medical care and medications before you need them.
- Understand the common medical illnesses and their treatments before you go (such as malaria, diarrhea, animal bites).
- If possible, take a friend with you when you visit the doctor who can help tell the doctor your history and question the doctor about the diagnosis and treatment.
- Try to avoid injections, or at least check out the needle before it enters your body.
- Carry adequate medical insurance.

There really isn't anything that will guarantee your health and safety, but traveling prepared and carrying adequate medical and travel insurance will make life easier should anything go wrong.

FIRST AID

Before I answer that often-asked question *"What medicines and supplies should I take along?"* let me say a bit about first aid and self-treatment. A complete guide to first aid is beyond the scope of this book, but that doesn't mean you should go to the other end of the world without a basic knowledge of how to deal with common medical problems. You do not need a medical degree, but it would be helpful to know the approach to things such as fevers, cuts and scrapes, head injuries, broken bones, burns, sprains, skin infections, bites, nosebleeds, allergic reactions, rashes, heat and cold injuries, seizures and much more!

So if you are planning a trip where anything can happen and you might not have or want access to local medical care, buy a first aid kit and a simple guide (that might come with your first aid kit), take a course or see what the Mayo Clinic recommends (www.mayoclinic.com/health/FirstAidIndex/FirstAidIndex).

Now back to the question, *"What medicines and supplies should I take along?"* My first suggestion to most people is to visit your medicine cabinet and see what you normally keep handy around the house. Then consider how far you'll be from decent medical care. You may need to take along what you would normally get at the drugstore or emergency department. Will you be responsible for others, such as your children, your students, fellow climbers or a tour group? Then you had better anticipate their needs as well.

There are many excellent commercially available first aid kits. They can usually be personalized for your specific needs. If you're contemplating minor surgery, consider taking a kit which contains sterile supplies such as syringes, needles and suture material. This would be appropriate for someone traveling off the beaten path, someone who is responsible for a group of travelers or anyone who distrusts needles around the world. While this sort of kit may be of help if you need an injection or a few stitches, it will not bail you out of a serious car accident or a ruptured appendix.

The following is a brief list of some of the more common and useful things to take along. (The brand names given here are not the only ones available.) Remember, what you take along will depend upon your particular situation.

SUGGESTED MEDICATIONS AND SUPPLIES

- altitude sickness (Diamox®, Adalat®, dexamethasone)
- analgesics/painkillers (acetaminophen, ASA, ibuprofen, codeine, Tylenol 3® or other narcotics)
- antacid/ulcers (Maalox®, Zantac®, Losec®)
- antibiotics (amoxicillin, cephalexin, erythromycin, ciprofloxacin, azithromycin)
- antidiarrheal (Imodium®, Lomotil®, Pepto-Bismol®)
- antifungal cream (Canesten®, Monistat®, Loprox®)
- antihistamine (Benadryl®)
- antimalarials (discuss with medical professional)
- antinauseant/motion sickness (Gravol®, Bonamine®, Phenergan®, Transderm V®/Transderm Scop® patches)
- bee sting kit (EpiPen®, Twinject®) for those with a history of severe allergic reactions
- cream/pills for vaginal infections (Monistat®, Diflucan®)
- eye drops (10% Sodium Sulamyd, Garamycin®)
- an extra pair of glasses or contact lenses and/or a copy of your prescription
- laxatives (Senokot®, Dulcolax®) — not everyone gets just diarrhea
- rehydration salts (Gastrolyte®, Pedialyte®)
- sunscreen
- topical antibiotic (Polysporin®, Fucidin®, Bactroban®)
- topical cortisone cream (Celestoderm®, 1% HC)

- other prescription and nonprescription medications used regularly
- adhesive tape
- antiseptic (Betadine®)
- Band-Aids®
- first aid guide
- flashlight and batteries
- gauze rolls
- insect repellent
- medical records and/or MedicAlert® bracelet
- moleskin
- mosquito net (preferably impregnated with permethrin)
- safety pins
- scissors
- sewing supplies
- small alarm clock
- sterile dressings
- sterile needles, suture supplies (Steri Aid Kit®)
- Steri-strips®
- Swiss Army knife
- tensor bandage
- thermometer
- toilet paper
- triangular bandage (sling)
- tweezers
- waterproof matches
- water purifier, iodine tablets, Pristine®

Chapter 2

THE JOYS OF TRAVEL

Wilbur Wright made the first flight on December 17, 1903. It lasted 12 seconds and spanned 120 feet. Hardly long enough to develop jet lag or a blood clot, catch the flu, complain about the food or lose your baggage! Things have changed, and now all of these things and more are possible. Let's discuss some of them.

GAS

As the airplane gains altitude and the ambient pressure in our pressurized aircraft becomes lower, the volume of any trapped gas in your body (e.g., sinuses and bowels) increases. This is known as Boyle's Law and it can lead to a couple of problems.

So as we eat and drink and sit bent at a right angle like a pretzel, and don't feel comfortable breaking wind, the gas that is trapped in our intestinal system expands, making us bloated and uncomfortable. Not the end of the world, but you might want to go easy on the beans and Brussels sprouts, and wear loose-fitting clothing with a few extra notches in the belt.

Air may also get trapped in our Eustachian tubes, the passageways leading to the eardrums from the nose, mouth and sinuses. This usually creates a problem during descent. As the pressure starts to increase, the trapped air contracts and creates a "sucking" effect on the eardrum. This may be quite painful and can lead to bleeding behind the eardrum. Those who are congested to start with may be particularly susceptible. To prevent or minimize this problem, try these measures:

- Drink, chew gum or swallow frequently as you descend.
- Breast-feed your baby if you have one.
- If you are already congested, take an oral or topical decongestant.
- Perform the Toynbee manoeuvre (pinch your nose, shut your mouth and blow) in order to re-expand your Eustachian tubes.
- Politely ask the pilot to perform a very gradual descent.

Other conditions where trapped gas might develop would be after laparoscopic surgery or a pneumothorax (the leakage of air around a lung). A recently applied plaster cast may also have gas bubbles which could expand during flight and make the cast dangerously tight. Seek medical attention if you think these conditions apply to you.

ECONOMY CLASS SYNDROME

Imagine sitting screwed up like the aforementioned pretzel for 12 hours. Welcome to long haul flights, and even some long drives. This common situation may predispose you to developing a blood clot or DVT (deep vein thrombosis) in the leg. The clot can break off and travel to the lung, causing a pulmonary embolism, a potentially fatal condition. Thankfully this is a fairly uncommon event, and when it occurs, it usually does so in people with certain underlying risk factors, such as: pregnancy, obesity, cigarette smokers, use of estrogen (hormone replacement or the birth control pill), varicose veins, cancer and previous DVT or pulmonary embolus.

If you are at higher risk of DVT, and perhaps even if you aren't, consider the following:

- Stay well hydrated by drinking lots of water, and not too much coffee or alcohol.
- Request an aisle or bulkhead seat.
- Wiggle, stretch and get up and stroll from time to time while you are aloft.
- Wear elastic compression stockings and loose fitting clothing.
- Consider an injection of low molecular weight heparin prior to departure. Discuss this with your doctor.

FAINTING

"Is there a doctor on board?" This common announcement happens most often because a passenger has fainted. Sitting in the now familiar pretzel position for too long may cause blood to pool in our legs, rather than returning to our brain. Eating too much diverts some of the blood to our intestines, and alcohol causes our blood vessels to dilate. All this leads to a drop in blood pressure when you get up to go empty your distended bladder! Before fainting, victims are usually pale, sweaty and "fuzzy." This is the best time to lay them down and elevate their feet!

THE AIR UP THERE

It is difficult to get the airline industry and the flyer to agree on the quality of the air when aloft. What is indisputable is that if you put 300 people in an enclosed space (such as an airplane), many of whom are coughing and sneezing, some bacteria and viruses are bound to circulate! There have been scares of tuberculosis being transmitted on aircrafts, but this is highly unlikely. Here are a few ways you can reduce the chances of spending your vacation by the vaporizer:

- Wear a mask.
- Don't travel if you are ill.
- Cough and sneeze into your elbow or sleeve, not your hands (for everyone else's sake).
- Wash your hands frequently.
- Get vaccinated against influenza and pneumonia.

JET LAG

Whether you feel it or not, your body has several rhythms that fluctuate during the course of the day and night. These rhythms control functions such as your blood pressure, heart rate, digestion, thinking and wakefulness. Ideally, all these individual clocks work in harmony. We take it for granted that we generally get hungry at the same times every day, we are full of energy at certain times of the day and we are ready to put our head on the pillow at 10 o'clock each night. The time of night varies from person to person and does not necessarily mean that your clock is broken.

Jet lag occurs when our internal body clock becomes out of sync with the clock at our destination. Jet lag can occur after crossing as few as three time zones. For example, you may be rushing off to see the pyramids in Egypt just when your brain was expecting to crawl under the covers for some badly needed sleep. Or conversely, it may be time for lights out, and you're counting sheep because you can't get to sleep. This biological clock is controlled by the naturally occurring hormone, melatonin, which is secreted by our pineal gland in the brain. The levels of melatonin fluctuate with the amount of light passing through our eyes.

The symptoms of jet lag may include:

- difficulty falling asleep or staying asleep
- fatigue during the day
- irritability
- difficulty concentrating or remembering things
- loss of appetite and change in bowel movements

The severity may depend upon the direction of your travel (west to east is said to be worse than east to west), though I am sure I suffer less when I get "there" (more excitement and anticipation) than when I return home (more bills to pay and work). Older people tend to adjust less well than younger people, perhaps because their sleeping habits may not be that great to start with.

Like everything else in life, some people may be more susceptible than others. The duration of your jet lag may be about a day for every time zone (there are 24) you have recently crossed. The impact of this will depend upon whether you have to give a PowerPoint presentation the day after you get home, or can continue on with your retirement! Fortunately, traveling north-south is not a problem, though a 12-hour flight to Chile may still leave you a bit under the weather.

How can I try to prevent it?

There are a few remedies for jet lag. Unfortunately, some of them are either ineffective or impractical, or both. Let's take a look at them.

- **Argonne Anti-Jet-Lag Diet.** This diet allegedly helps travelers adjust their body clock to the new time zone. It involves manipulating your food intake, caffeine intake and proportions of protein and carbohydrates and timing, and in my opinion, is a bit complicated, to say the least. (www.antijetlagdiet. com).

- **Exposure to light** before you travel and upon your arrival at your destination. Light exposure has an effect upon the production of melatonin in the brain. Apparently, eastward travel requires exposure to bright light early in the day after arrival, and westward travel requires it at the end of the day.

- **Acupressure** involves balancing your meridian system by massaging specific pressure points regularly while traveling and upon arrival. The Jet Lag Eliminator will help you discover these points (www.jetlag.net).

- **No-Jet-Lag** is a homeopathic remedy containing arnica, bellis perennis, chamomilla, ipecacuanha and lycopodium. The tablets need to be taken at take-off, every two hours in flight and then after each landing (including at intermediate stops). Many people swear by this remedy and studies have suggested that it's effective, so consider giving it a try. (www.nojetlag.com)

- **Melatonin.** Levels of melatonin are lowest during the day when we are awake and exposed to lots of light, and highest at night—helping us sleep, we think. There are many studies supporting the use of melatonin for jet lag as well as other sleep disturbances. It supposedly works by causing a "chemical darkness."

    For eastward flight, it may be taken in the early evening for two or three days prior to departure.

Upon arrival, take it a bit later at the local bedtime for as many nights as it takes you to get properly adjusted to the local time. If you are going west, then melatonin may be used at bedtime at your destination.

The recommended dosage is between 3 and 5 milligrams. I am sure you will find other dosages and schedules if you look. Melatonin may cause some drowsiness and should not be used by the young and the pregnant. Those on anticoagulants and with epilepsy should also avoid it.

- **A short-acting sleeping pill or hypnotic** is a common request of travelers for use on the plane, as well as for a short time at their destination and/or when they return home. This does nothing to readjust the body's clock, but it may get you a decent night's sleep. Sleeping pills (e.g., zopiclone, temazepam, zolpidem) may cause drowsiness, and some people may have difficulty with their short-term memory when they wake up. In the elderly, these should be used cautiously or not at all.

I don't believe that jet lag is totally responsible for us feeling as bad as we sometimes do when we reach our destination. Imagine sitting in your den strapped into a narrow seat, constantly being served meals and cocktails, surrounded by screaming infants, and watching a six-inch screen as your bladder almost bursts for 12 hours! So here's some more advice that might come in handy.

- Fly business class if you can.
- Drink lots of fluids while in flight, preferably water. Avoid, or minimize, coffee and alcohol consumption. They cause dehydration and upset your sleep patterns. Try to sit near the lavatory!

- Don't eat everything that comes your way. Gases expand in the air up there. Your belt will need an extra notch or two by the time you arrive.
- Take a stretch or stroll every hour.
- If you fly at night, try to get some sleep on the plane. Use earplugs, a blindfold and an inflatable pillow.
- Switch to the local time schedule upon your arrival. A cold shower or a quick swim may invigorate you for the day ahead. Try to avoid napping during the day, and hit the sack at night, local time, when you're totally bushed.
- Schedule a one-night (or longer) stopover on your way if possible.

Jet lag and long flights are just some of the joys of travel, right up there with motion sickness, lost baggage and parking fees. Do what you can do, or want to do, to minimize it. It will soon pass!

SUN EXPOSURE

A tan is no longer a sign of good health. Rather, it means skin injury. As sunshine is ubiquitous, especially when we travel, we should be aware of its negative effects and how to minimize them.

What is it?

There are three types of ultraviolet radiation to which we are exposed:

1. **UVA** (320–400 nanometers) — This longer wave radiation is responsible for most photosensitivity reactions, and also contributes to chronic skin damage, sunburn and the risk of skin cancer. UVA levels stay relatively constant throughout the day and the year.

2. **UVB** (290–320 nanometers) — This middle wave radiation is the major cause of sunburn and chronic skin injury, including aging and skin cancer. UVB rays are most intense between 10 a.m. and 4 p.m. They can penetrate one meter of water, and are reflected 17 percent by water, 50 percent by sand and up to 80 percent by snow. At higher altitudes where the air is thinner (the Guatemalan highlands was my last sunburn site), these rays become much more intense.

3. **UVC** (less than 280 nanometers) — This range of radiation is blocked by the ozone layer and doesn't reach the earth's surface. However it is found in artificial light sources such as tanning beds.

Melanin is the chemical in our skin that protects our skin by reflecting and absorbing UV rays. Those who have less of it, i.e., those with lighter skin and red or blond hair are at greater risk. So are people with numerous moles or a family history of skin cancer. Commonly used medications such as doxycycline (an antimalarial), diuretics and sulfa may cause photosensitivity. Some unfortunate people are allergic to the sun, and quickly develop bumps, hives or blisters when exposed. Most of our harmful sun exposure occurs while we are young, so prevention is particularly crucial in children. UV radiation is also bad for the eyes by increasing the risk of cataracts.

There are three types of skin cancer — basal cell carcinomas, squamous cell carcinomas and malignant melanomas. While the latter is the least common, it is by far the most deadly. All forms of skin cancer are increaseing.

Sunburn, which I suppose is our immediate concern when we travel, can be extremely uncomfortable and debilitating, and might throw off your vacation more than a wicked case of the runs!

How do we prevent sun damage?

There are a number of measures that should be taken so that you don't leave the beach looking like a lobster, or spend your golden years in the dermatologist's office.

1. Stay away from tanning salons. Evidence suggests that the use of tanning beds before the age of 30 increases the risk of skin cancer by 75 percent. They have recently been placed in the same cancer-risk category as arsenic and mustard gas!
2. Minimize your sun exposure between 10 a.m. and 4 p.m. UV rays can penetrate the clouds so don't be lulled into a false sense of security just because of the overcast sky or the refreshing breeze.
3. Babies under six months of age should be kept out of direct sunlight.
4. Wear protective clothing. Tightly woven fabrics are preferable. Wear a hat.

5. Wear sunglasses, preferably of the wraparound variety. Not all lenses are created equal, so read the fine print.
6. Use sunscreen or sunblock or both.

How to choose and use sunscreen:

- Choose a sunscreen that is "broad spectrum," i.e., provides protection against both UVA and UVB rays, and preferably one that is water and sweat resistant.
- Apply it generously about 20 minutes before going out. Don't forget those more obscure areas like your ears, nose and tops of your feet. Sunblocks, like zinc oxide and titanium dioxide, are ideal for these areas, and they are available in a rainbow of pleasing colors.
- Reapply it every two hours, and more often if you are sweating a lot or swimming.
- Pick a sunscreen with an SPF (sun protection factor) of at least 15. If you are one of those sensitive people, pick a higher SPF. The higher that number, theoretically the longer you will be protected.
- With children, mom or dad should do the applying, taking care to avoid the eyes, mouth and fingers.
- If there are insect-borne infections around (e.g., dengue fever) or just irritating bugs, use an insect repellent as well, which should be applied about 20 minutes after your sunscreen.

Sunburn can be treated with analgesics such as aspirin, ibuprofen, perhaps an antihistamine such as diphenhydramine (Benadryl®) and cool baths or compresses. Topical medications such as cortisone or menthol may help as well. Blisters should be left intact if possible and topical anesthetics such as Lanacane® should be avoided. More severe burns may require further medical attention.

MOTION SICKNESS

To travel means to be on the move, whether it be by land, air or sea. And one of the dangers of movement is motion sickness, an unpleasant and sometimes embarrassing condition. Julius Caesar was nauseated in his chariot and many astronauts have experienced it, so don't be surprised if it happens to you.

What is motion sickness?

Motion sickness is an unfortunate condition arising from information overload to your inner ear and brain — too many conflicting signals. While bumpy roads, choppy waters and turbulent air are more likely to make you sick, it can occur even when things are relatively calm. It may be rather humbling as you feel stomach discomfort, nausea, drowsiness, lightheadedness and the need to gasp for air and to sigh. People around you notice that you are pale and sweaty. Eventually, these feelings may culminate in an uncontrollable desire to throw up.

For most people, motion sickness will be only a slight nuisance, but for others it may take a few days to adapt. Some unlucky souls actually experience the same thing when they get back onto dry land, as they readjust to their new reality. Children aged 2 to 12 are the most susceptible, along with those who have experienced it before (like me!).

How can I prevent it?

Well you can avoid rough waters, lousy roads and turbulent flights, and if that doesn't work, try the following:

- Choose the best available seat; in a car, that would be the front passenger or driver's seat; in a boat, somewhere in the middle; and on a plane, over the wing (but inside the plane).

- Avoid big meals, alcohol and cigarette smoke.
- Refrain from reading.
- Focus on distant objects like the horizon or the TV screen.
- Before you depart, consider taking along medications such as diphenhydrinate (Gravol®), meclizine (Bonamine®), a scopolamine patch (Transderm-Scop® or Transderm-V®). The patch may cause drowsiness, blurred vision or difficulty urinating, so try them before you leave).
- Try ginger root (*Zingiber officinale*), as capsules, lozenges or in the dry root form.
- Try Trip Ease®, a homeopathic concoction.
- Try acupressure, a small bracelet worn around the wrist, such as the Sea-Band.

What if you get it?

The ideal treatment is to get off your moving vehicle, be it plane, train, boat or automobile. If that is not possible, move to a more desirable location, and stare at the horizon. Medications might or might not be a bit late at this point.

ALTITUDE SICKNESS

Many of the world's most popular destinations are situated at high altitudes, that is, above 7,500 feet. Coming down with altitude sickness may be no worse than your last hangover or tension headache. On the other hand, it can prove fatal. So if your dream is to trek to Everest Base Camp, explore the ruins of Machu Picchu, paddle on Lake Titicaca, visit the temples in Lhasa or scale Kilimanjaro, this chapter is for you.

What is altitude sickness?

As we ascend above 7,500 feet or so, the amount of oxygen in the air decreases, so we have less oxygen for our red blood cells to deliver to vital organs such as our lungs and brain. This relative lack of oxygen is called "hypoxia." Our body does its best to compensate for this effect by immediately increasing the heart rate and respiratory rate and, within a few weeks, producing more red blood cells. Just about everyone in this situation will feel some shortness of breath and a pounding heart, but this is not really altitude sickness. **Acute mountain sickness (AMS)** is usually the first and mildest form of altitude sickness, and one might experience such hangover-like symptoms as a throbbing headache, nausea, vomiting, loss of appetite, dizziness and insomnia. It will usually begin within 24 hours of arrival at high altitude. Your likelihood of developing AMS may depend on a few things, such as:

- How high you go.
- How quickly you go high.
- How warm and hydrated you stay.
- Your own personal predisposition to altitude sickness.

It does not depend on your age or fitness level. Seniors often do better at high altitudes because they are more patient, or forced to go slower. Most at risk are the triathletes who want to scamper up the mountain, or are too stubborn to pay attention to their headaches. Most people will successfully acclimatize and feel better, but the key is, if you continue to ascend with symptoms of AMS, it may lead to the more serious forms of altitude sickness, such as the following:

High altitude pulmonary edema (HAPE) occurs when the pressure in our pulmonary (lung) arteries increases and the blood vessels become leaky, causing fluid (edema) to build up in our lungs. This may lead to fatigue, coughing and shortness of breath, not just with exertion but also when we are at rest. Breathing is usually worse at night when lying flat. Many people will experience "periodic breathing" at night — the annoying sensation that you can't get enough breath. This is not dangerous, but it's not conducive to a restful sleep.

High altitude cerebral edema (HACE) is also caused by leaky blood vessels that cause swelling of the brain. It may start with a severe headache, some confusion or a change in behavior. Unsteadiness is characteristic, and coma and death will follow if not properly treated, and quickly!

High altitude retinopathy refers to the small hemorrhages that may occur at the back of the eye (retina) at altitudes above 15,000 feet. Depending on a hemorrhage's location on the retina, vision may or may not be affected. This condition usually resolves itself within 10 to 14 days.

High altitude flatus expulsion, if you must know, occurs because trapped gases expand at lower pressures (i.e., at higher altitudes). Hence, a little bit more bloating and farting may be expected!

Where do we get it?

The following table shows the altitudes of the most common

high-altitude destinations. Remember though, it's not just the altitude. Other factors are involved, such as how quickly you ascend, whether you stop to acclimatize at higher altitudes and how warm and well hydrated you stay.

Mexico City	7,349 ft. / 2,240 m
Aspen, Colorado	7,890 ft. / 2,405 m
Bogotá, Colombia	8,661 ft. / 2,640 m
Quito, Ecuador	9,350 ft. / 2,850 m
Cuzco, Peru	11,200 ft. / 3,400 m
La Paz, Bolivia	11,942 ft. / 3,640 m
Lhasa, Tibet	11,450 ft. / 3,490 m
Mount Kinabalu, Malaysia	13,435 ft. / 4,095 m
Everest South Base Camp, Nepal	17,600 ft. / 5,360 m
Mount Kilimanjaro, Tanzania	19,334 ft. / 5,893 m
Mount Logan, Yukon	19,551 ft. / 5,959 m
Mount McKinley, Alaska	20,320 ft. / 6,193 m
Mount Aconcagua, Argentina	22,841 ft. / 6,962 m
Mount Everest, Nepal	29,029 ft. / 8,848 m

Kilimanjaro is one of the more dangerous and difficult destinations, because climbers typically ascend it in five or six days. This rate of ascent exceeds the 1,000–1,500-foot change in your sleeping altitude that is recommended. Getting to Everest South Base Camp usually takes a few weeks, a much safer and more gradual ascent. The trek to Machu Picchu reaches almost 14,000 feet (4,267 meters) at Dead Woman's Pass, but is downhill from there. Flying to either La Paz, Bolivia, or Lhasa, Tibet, usually involves an abrupt ascent that may bring on symptoms of AMS.

How do we prevent it?

There are a number of things that can be done to reduce the

likelihood of developing altitude sickness, including:

- Go slow, go slow, go slow ... or "*Pole, pole, pole,*" as your Kilimanjaro guides will tell you.
- Drink plenty of water ... enough to keep your urine clear.
- Avoid alcohol and other depressants, such as sleeping pills.
- Don't ascend more than 1,500 feet per day.
- If possible, every three days spend a day resting to acclimatize.
- Dress warmly.
- Try the local remedies like coca tea or garlic soup. Gingko biloba has not been shown to work.
- Climb high ... sleep low – it's the sleeping altitude that counts.
- It is very important not to ascend higher if you have symptoms of altitude sickness.
- Consider using acetazolamide (Diamox®) preventively.
- Some more-driven climbers have been known to use dexamethasone (Decadron®) to ensure they get to the top — 4 mg every 12 hours.

A word about Diamox®. This is a useful medication that works by increasing the acidity of your blood. In response, your body breathes more quickly and blows off more carbon dioxide, or hyperventilates. This in turn provides more oxygen, which is what you are missing at higher altitudes and what your system would get if given the time. Diamox® does not mask the symptoms of altitude sickness; it prevents them by speeding up your acclimatization.

Diamox® is related to sulfa and should probably be avoided by those with a sulfa allergy, though this suggestion may be a bit controversial. It may cause a few bothersome side effects

– you may pee a bit more, your fingers and toes may tingle, and beer and carbonated drinks will taste a bit funny. But it will help prevent those headaches and fitful nights.

The dosage of Diamox® in adults is 125 mg (usually half a pill) twice a day, and it can be started the day before your ascent. It could then be continued during your entire stay at high altitude, or discontinued at some point. Children may also take Diamox® in the appropriate dosage (5 mg/kg a day).

Certain travelers should probably stay closer to sea level, including those with angina, congestive heart failure or chronic obstructive pulmonary disease. Hypertension and asthma should not be any worse up high, though asthma is sometimes aggravated by exertion or cold air. Sickle cell disease and severe anemia from any cause are two more reasons to stay put. And finally, pregnant women would be advised not to spend much time over 12,000 feet, partly because of the thinner air, but also because medical care is not always the best at many of these destinations.

What if you get it?

There is a quote attributable to Dr. David Shlim: *"It's OK to get altitude sickness, but it's not OK to die from it."* So read closely.

Mild AMS can usually be treated with rest, simple pain-killers such as aspirin or acetaminophen, lots of fluids, and perhaps Diamox®. Symptoms should resolve quickly, and if they don't, it would be best to descend at least 500 feet or to the last altitude at which you felt well, or seek out some oxygen. If your headache does not stop, the last thing you want to do is start climbing higher. Zofran® (ondansetron) is a useful medication to treat the nausea of AMS.

HACE and HAPE are medical emergencies, and the treatment should include at least some of the following:

- **Descent**, as mentioned before, of at least 500 feet (152 meters), or to good medical care if necessary.

- **Oxygen** if it's available.
- **Minimal exertion** (stay warm).
- **Nifedipine (Adalat®)** — 20 mg by mouth and repeated every six hours for the treatment of HAPE.
- **Dexamethasone (Decadron®)** — 8 mg intramuscularly or by mouth and then 4 mg every six hours for the treatment of HACE. This decreases swelling in the brain, rather than aiding acclimatization. Rebound symptoms may occur if medication is discontinued. Don't ascend again unless you have been off of the medication for at least a day.
- **Hyperbaric oxygen (e.g., Gamow)** — an airtight sleeping bag that may be pressurized by means of a simple foot pump. The increased pressure in the bag simulates descent and improves the amount of oxygen available to the sufferer. Most climbers do not have this $2,000 piece of equipment; if you do, it should be used only to buy time, not as a substitute for descent. It may not be suitable for someone who is claustrophobic or comatose.

HACE and HAPE are not always predictable or preventable, but in most cases serious forms of altitude sickness are preceded by more subtle signs. Denial may be a big problem up there. Early recognition and treatment are the keys to safe climbing.

Altitude sickness may affect anyone — the young or the elderly, male or female, and those both in and out of shape. If you have suffered from it before, you may be more prone the next time as well. So go slowly, drink that water, put on your sunscreen and sunglasses, consider the use of Diamox® and enjoy the most breathtaking views of your life.

TRAVELER'S DIARRHEA

They say *"Travel expands the mind ... and loosens the bowels,"* and most people who have visited the tropics or lesser-developed countries know why! Up to 40 percent of visitors to these destinations will suffer some intestinal upset, usually diarrhea. For many, it is just an inconvenience, but for some it will be severe enough to ruin your trip or land you in the local medical facility. More colorful names for this condition include Delhi Belly, Montezuma's Revenge and Seeping Slickness!

What is Traveler's Diarrhea?

It may be self evident, but for the record, the scientific definition of Traveler's Diarrhea (TD) is *"passing three or more unformed bowel movements within 24 hours."* It may be much more! Other symptoms that may add to your suffering include fever and chills, abdominal cramps, aches and pains and vomiting. If there is blood or mucus in your stools, this is known as dysentery, which may be from an ameba or various bacteria. If TD is severe and not properly treated, dehydration occurs and hospital treatment is required. Small children are more susceptible to this.

The following table shows you the various causes of TD. The majority of infections contracted abroad are bacterial infections. Of that bunch, *Enterotoxigenic E. coli* is probably responsible for at least 50 percent of cases. It usually causes a relatively mild, self-limited bout of diarrhea. It follows the "rule of threes" — starts on the third day of your trip, consists of three loose bowel movements per day, and lasts about three days. *Enteroaggretive E. coli* causes a similar illness.

Other bacteria such as *Salmonella*, *Shigella* and *Campylobacter*, on the other hand, can make you much sicker, sometimes with dysentery. *Clostridium difficile* is a ubiquitous bacterium that occasionally infects those who

CAUSES OF TRAVELER'S DIARRHEA

Bacterial

Enterotoxigenic E. coli

Enteroaggretive E. coli

Salmonella

Shigella

Campylobacter

Clostridium difficile

Vibrio cholera

Protozoal

Amebiasis

Giardiasis

Cyclosporiasis

Crptosporidiosis

Viral

Norovirus

Rotavirus

Non-infectious

Inflammatory bowel disease

Lactose intolerance

Tropical sprue

Celiac disease

Hyperthyroidism

Irritable bowel syndrome

Colon cancer

have been on antibiotics for another condition. It is capable of causing severe diarrhea and dysentery. Finally, infection with *Vibrio cholera*, the cause of cholera, may result in profuse watery diarrhea leading to dehydration and death. It tends to occur in outbreaks (in Zimbabwe most recently) and is an exceedingly rare cause of diarrhea in travelers.

Parasites account for a small proportion of TD. Infection with *Giardia lamblia* or giardiasis (AKA beaver fever) is well known for causing chronic diarrhea, along with gas, bloating, rumbling and farts that will curl your nose. Milk products may run through you because of associated lactose intolerance. *Entameba histolytica* can cause mild to severe diarrhea, and sometimes dysentery. As well, it can spread to your liver and create an abscess. There are several other amebas but they usually cause mild or no illness. *Crytosporidium* and *Cyclospora* are two less common parasites that are capable of causing more severe and longer lasting diarrhea.

Viruses are responsible for about 20 percent of cases of TD. Norovirus (Norwalk virus) is well known for causing virulent outbreaks of vomiting and diarrhea on cruise ships. Intestinal worms, such as roundworms and hookworms, are abundant in the tropics, but are rarely contracted by tourists and likely won't cause diarrhea anyway.

Finally, just a change in your diet, fruit or alcohol intake or time zone may be enough to alter your usual bowel patterns.

There are several ways to get TD. They include:

- Drinking contaminated water (this includes ice cubes).
- Eating uncooked or undercooked food that has been contaminated.
- Eating food that has been poorly refrigerated or has sat out in the sun for too long.

- Eating food that has been contaminated by flies.
- Having close contact, e.g., shaking hands with someone or touching a doorknob that is infected.

Some people may be more susceptible to getting TD, such as those immunosuppressed with HIV/AIDS or on acid-blocking medications.

Where do we get it?

Traveler's Diarrhea is more likely to occur in the tropics in association with poverty. While sanitary conditions have improved over the years in tourist destinations such as Mexico, Cuba and the Dominican Republic, TD is still common. The Indian subcontinent might have the highest risk. Egypt seems to produce a high number of cases as do the poorer parts of Latin America. Anything goes in sub-Saharan Africa. The shorter your stay and the more precautions you take, the less likely you will be spending extra time on the toilet!

A few generalizations:

- There might be greater access to safe food and water in big cities.
- A five star (or more) restaurant is probably safer than no stars or the local market.
- The quality of the food and water might be proportional to the degree of local poverty.
- The rainy season might result in more food and water-borne disease.
- You are only as safe as the last person who handled your food.

How do we prevent it?

If you adhere to the mantra *"Boil it, bottle it, peel it, cook it or forget it,"* and wash your hands, your chances of becoming ill will be much less. Here are some basic precautions:

- Bring your water to a rolling boil for a minute or two; much longer and you'll run out of water and fuel! Above 6,000 feet, boil for three minutes.
- Buy bottled water, but check that the seal has not been tampered with.
- Treat your water with iodine (tincture of iodine two percent solution, add five drops to a liter of clear water. If the water is cloudy, add 10 drops per liter. The resultant taste can be eliminated with some vitamin C or juice crystals). Pristine® (chlorine dioxide) leaves no aftertaste and is also effective against *Cryptosporidium.*
- Use a water purification system. These usually employ a combination of a filter and iodine (e.g., PUR®, Katadyn®, MSR® and First Need®) and come in numerous sizes and shapes.
- Drink carbonated drinks, beer or wine.
- Eat food that has been cooked, well-cooked, and in the case of street food, has been cooked in front of your own eyes; this means that you might avoid salads.
- Peel your fruits.
- Uncooked veggies can be soaked in a solution of chlorine (bleach) or permanganate, and rinsed with clean water.
- Wash your hands frequently, and take along a hand sanitizer such as Purell®.
- Make sure you don't swallow any of the water when you have a shower.
- Take Dukoral® prior to your trip. This oral vaccine will reduce your chance of contracting diarrhea from *Enterotoxigenic E. coli* by about 60 percent

and overall by about 30 percent. If you are truly at risk of cholera (e.g., working in a disaster situation) consider it as well.

- Higher risk, shorter term travelers (e.g., underlying inflammatory bowel disease, President of the Free World) might consider a prophylactic antibiotic such as ciprofloxacin (Cipro®) or rifaximin (Xifaxan®).

The above measures do not guarantee a cramp-free holiday. How closely you adhere to the above list will depend upon your individual surroundings, your budget and your level of paranoia. For longer term and higher risk travelers, TD is probably inevitable at some point.

What if you get it?

The treatment of TD depends upon how sick you are, and your individual tolerance for being sick. Here are the basics:

- **Oral rehydration therapy** with ORS (oral rehydration salts) or other homemade clear fluids such as soup with salt or tea with sugar; Pedialyte® or Gastrolyte® are great; rice or cereal based ORS is also available. Then progress onto bland foods such as rice, boiled potatoes and bananas. Children can probably be kept on their regular solids if willing. You can make your own ORS by mixing 1 teaspoon of salt, 8 teaspoons of sugar and 4 ounces of orange juice (optional) mixed into 1 liter of clean water.
- **Antiperistaltics**, such as loperamide (Imodium®), slow the movement of things through your intestine, that is, they relieve some of your discomfort. Use these in small quantities, perhaps one-half or one pill, lest you never go to the bathroom again. This should not be used alone if you have fever or blood in your

stools or if you would prefer to let those things get out of you. They should not be taken by small children or pregnant women.

- **Bismuth subsalicylate** (Pepto Bismol®) may be helpful for mild cases.
- **Antibiotics**, such as ciprofloxacin (Cipro®) and azithromycin (Zithromax®) are extremely useful, given that bacteria are responsible for most cases of acute diarrhea. Azithromycin is more appropriate for kids under 16, pregnant women and travelers to Southeast Asia. The usual antibiotic course is for three days, but if you are better in a day or two, the antibiotic can be stopped. Antibiotics may be used with a small amount of loperamide. Not everyone with diarrhea needs an antibiotic, but if you are quite sick (fever, frequent bowel movements, blood or pus in the stools), are not getting better, or just want a quicker recovery, they can be very effective.
- **Rifaximin** (Xifaxan®) is a relatively new, non-absorbable antibiotic used to treat "non-invasive" diarrhea, which is usually caused by ETEC (*Enterotoxigenic E. coli*). It can be used over the age of 12, but currently is not available in Canada.
- **Antiparasitics**, such as metronidazole or tinidazole, can be taken if you are suspected of harboring an intestinal parasite.
- **Natural remedies** such as probiotics (*acidophilus, lactobacillus, bifidobacterium, saccharomyces*), charcoal, garlic, oregano or grapefruit seed extract may be of help.

Chapter 3

CULTURE SHOCK & PERSONAL SAFETY

WHAT IS CULTURE SHOCK?

Imagine being dropped in a foreign land where the language was incomprehensible, the people dressed differently, the food was unrecognizable, it was 100°F / 37.7°C in the shade, you had no friends and the water was always cold … that is, when there was water. Now imagine staying there for a year. It might be a bit disconcerting at times, don't you think? So let's talk about culture shock and your mental health. Most of what follows pertains to longer-term travelers or expatriates rather than to one-week resort tourists.

Culture shock is an interesting syndrome brought on by the stress that results from the loss of all or many of our familiar signs, symbols and surroundings — the things we have taken for granted for many years — and plunging into something totally different. We go from English, hot water, high-speed Internet, 24-hour electricity and 20 varieties of bagels and coffee to a completely new environment. We are like fish out of water. We have all had this experience before, though in a mild way — perhaps when we moved homes, went away to college, changed jobs or met a new boyfriend or girlfriend. But it undoubtedly will be a lot more pronounced when we change cultures.

There are three classical stages to culture shock, and not everyone goes through them to the same extent or at the same rate or at all.

Stage 1 or the "honeymoon phase." *Wow, isn't this fantastic. I love the food, we've met some fantastic people, everyone is so friendly and I can't wait to get started at my new job. What a great move it was to come here.*

Stage 2 or the "oy vay stage." *My volunteer placement isn't working out, I hate the food, wish I could speak Swahili, I have diarrhea, I miss my dog and I wish there was a Starbucks nearby. I'm feeling pretty frustrated and sometimes run out of patience, and water. What am I doing here? Time for another beer!*

Stage 3 or the "I'm lovin' it stage." *My Swahili isn't bad. I think I'm making a difference in the program. I kind of like the local food and have made some great friends. The cold showers are refreshing. The kids are great. Wish I could stay longer … maybe I will!*

It's that second stage you need to worry about. You may not just be frustrated, but also quite negative and even anxious or depressed. These feelings may in turn affect your mood, your energy levels, sleep patterns, sex drive and appetite. Your sense of humor, perhaps your most valuable asset, may disappear.

How can you prevent it?

It may not be necessary to "prevent" something that may be quite natural and expected. Here are some steps you can take to ease your transition into another culture.

- Realize that culture shock may occur.
- Learn as much as you can about your new home before you leave.
- Take some time to acclimatize to the jet lag, the food, the living conditions and the weather.
- Have realistic expectations. You may have plans to change the world; just don't expect to do it all in the first week.
- Commit yourself to learning the local language.
- Keep in touch with friends and family and with events back home.
- Make the most of your work. Set small, realistic goals and try to tolerate what you cannot change. This shift in attitude may be quite difficult if it involves tolerating things you wouldn't accept at home, like corruption, corporal punishment, poor treatment of women and other customs and behaviors.
- Make use of and offer peer support.
- Deal with stress as it arises. Learn how to deal with stress before you need to. Study yoga or meditation before you leave.
- If you have time available, use it to get in shape, develop a new skill, travel, volunteer and discover the culture.
- If you've brought children along, take advantage of the time you spend together.
- Be proactive about your health. Pay attention to diet and hygiene, and get regular rest, exercise and relaxation.
- Take along some special things from home — your favorite photos, an iPod with 3,000 songs, packaged teas, duty-free chocolate, etc. — and enjoy them when you're feeling lonely or blue.
- Ask for help if you need it.

What if you get it?

It's not just the problem of culture shock. Anxiety and depression can occur in anyone at any time. They happen all of the time in the Western world, so why not where you end up? There may be the impression among your friends and family that, if you are going to work or volunteer in a foreign country, you will be escaping all of life's stresses. Not true. You may just be exposed to new ones, like loneliness, job frustration, corruption, harassment, illness and much more. Or, it may be heaven on earth!

So the first step is to be aware that these problems can occur, and try to recognize them in yourself or others if they do. Be aware of the symptoms of depression:

- lack of energy and motivation
- changes in your eating and sleeping patterns
- irritability
- trouble concentrating
- feeling low or blue and being unable to enjoy things
- feeling worthless or guilty
- thoughts of suicide

Alcohol use may make things worse, and there may be a tendency to drink more when you are abroad (beer may be cheap, and it's cold and sterile). You may be bored or subject to peer pressure, and a drink may help you forget your problems and feelings. It may also dangerously lower your inhibitions. Drink responsibly!

What qualities will I need when I travel abroad?

Undoubtedly, you'll need many qualities if you're going to manage successfully when you are away from home — whether you travel for pleasure or work, and whether you're gone for a week or a year. Which one is most important? That probably depends on the person and the situation, but one volunteer I met was adamant that a sense of humor is paramount. *"If you can't laugh about some of the things that go on, you will have to cry."*

Here are some of the qualities you will need: open-mindedness, a sense of humor, an ability to cope with failure, communicativeness, flexibility and adaptability, curiosity, positive and realistic expectations, tolerance for differences and ambiguities, a positive regard for others, and a strong sense of self.

How about reverse culture shock?

You've just returned home after 12 glorious months in rural Nepal. You made great friends, had a wonderful job, loved the dal bhat and got to enjoy the cold showers. But isn't it great to see your old friends and family? Walk the dog. Go out to Starbucks. Have high-speed Internet! Well it may be great for a while … again a honeymoon phase. But once the reality sets in that everyone else has moved on with their lives, you miss your simple way of life; you're living in your parents' basement without a job and you don't know what the future holds—you may feel a little bit down and frustrated.

This transition can in fact be more difficult on coming home than going "over there." But realize that, with time, you will reintegrate into your old way of life. When excitedly showing your buddies a thousand of your favorite photos, remember to take the time to ask about what's been going on in their lives. As well, keep in touch with your new friends overseas. Offer to give a talk about your experiences. Look after your physical health and be patient. Sometimes counseling is in order. But given time, things will work out.

PERSONAL SAFETY

We spend a lot of time talking about exotic and not-so-exotic tropical diseases, while in fact they account for only a small fraction of the serious illness and death in travelers. Personal injuries, on the other hand, play a significant role. When my children and patients travel, I really don't worry so much about tropical infections, which are usually either preventable or manageable. Rather, I lie awake at night thinking of them riding in those buses on those roads.

Several studies have focused on the causes of death in travelers. The breakdown goes something like this:

- **Medical illnesses** such as heart attacks and strokes account for about two-thirds of the deaths in travelers. Older travelers are at greatest risk. This is not unlike the situation back home, where these illnesses are the major causes of mortality.
- **Infectious diseases**, such as malaria, typhoid fever, rabies and hepatitis, typically account for less than three percent of deaths abroad. Talking about these infectious risks, however, probably takes up about 90 percent of the time you spend with the doctor before you leave.
- **Trauma** consistently accounts for at least 25 percent of the deaths abroad. This more often involves young travelers, and more often males than females. The latter finding may be because males are more prone to taking risks, or that they are just not as intelligent as females. Probably a bit of both. The nature of these deaths tends to vary from country to country. Of this 25 percent, the greatest cause of death is motor vehicle accidents — cars, motorbikes, buses, tro-tros, matatus … you name it. The Peace Corps stopped allowing their volunteers to ride

motorbikes several years ago. Homicide, drowning, electrocution, suicide, poisoning and avalanches are some other gruesome causes.

RULES OF THE ROAD

It's not surprising that motor vehicle accidents are particularly high on the list of causes of death among travelers. Here are some of the reasons. They are generalizations, and not meant to offend those in the transportation business abroad.

- Cars and buses may be poorly maintained (missing dashboards, rear-view mirrors, seatbelts and more).
- Vehicles don't usually leave the station until they are packed — really packed!
- The drivers may be underage, intoxicated, or both, and are motivated to get from point A to point B with as many people as possible and as quickly as possible.
- The roads are poorly lit and lack white lines down the center.
- Potholes the size of swimming pools abound and everyone must do their best to avoid them, often at the same time coming from different directions.
- The sides of the roads are busy with people, baboons and cattle.
- The roads may be tortuous with steep cliffs on one side and no barriers.

For better or for worse, you can't always avoid the local form of transportation. Often there is no other practical choice. And what better way to see the country and its people than by staying on the ground. But please give some consideration to the following:

- Avoid driving at night in rural areas.

- If traveling by bus, try to find the best one you can afford.
- Stay off motorbikes if at all possible; get some proper training if you will be riding one regularly.
- Don't drink and drive, and don't drive with someone who has been drinking.
- At least look for a seatbelt.
- If you are taking along young children, make sure you arrange for a proper car seat.
- Use a local driver when possible. This decision may depend on the amount of confidence you have in the local driver versus yourself.
- Sitting in the back seat is statistically safer than in the front seat.
- Choose your taxi with care. Anecdotes abound of unsuspecting travelers being driven to remote spots, robbed and left on the roadside.
- The traffic may be going in the "wrong" direction. Look carefully before crossing the street.
- Avoid driving at night in rural areas. (Yes, I'm mentioning it again. It's important!)

DON'T GET MUGGED

Now that I've frightened you out of getting into a moving vehicle while you're away, let's talk about how you can avoid getting mugged, robbed and worse? My intention is not to make you paranoid and distrustful, but rather to make you aware of what may be going on around you.

Here are some tips to help you avoid unwanted trouble. Many apply particularly to women. The list is long, but it's based on the anecdotes of many unfortunate travelers over the years. Pick the points that apply to you:

- Leave your jewelry at home.

- Leave any valuables in the hotel safe, if there is one.
- Make copies of your passport and other important documents. Keep one copy with you and leave one at home.
- Carry a few extra passport photos. They might come in handy.
- Don't carry a purse. If you must, keep it close to your body, not dangling by a long strap.
- Change your traveler's checks and money only at "licensed" establishments. Count your money inside, not as you walk out the front door. Be vigilant at ATMs.
- Don't carry large amounts of money.
- If you are wearing a money belt, it's best to have it concealed under your clothing around your waist. Don't keep one around your ankle or neck.
- Buy a jacket that has zipper pockets.
- Divide your money and valuables among different pockets.
- Do not let your bags out of your sight. What gets stored on the top of the bus may not be there at the end of your 12-hour ride. When on a train, or anywhere else, do not leave your bags unattended.
- Be aware of your surroundings at all times. Be especially vigilant around markets, airports, and train and bus stations. If all of a sudden there are eight people surrounding you, something may be going on. Get yourself out of there as quickly as possible.
- Be sensitive to the local culture. Dress appropriately and perhaps somewhat conservatively. You already look like a wealthy tourist without making it more obvious.
- Don't try to photograph any sensitive buildings. They can usually be identified by the armed guards out front.

- Be tactful when it comes to taking pictures of local people. Some cultures do not allow it. Others just don't like it. Be sure you have "implied consent" before snapping away.
- Be alert to scams (*"Oh, I'm sorry. I seem to have dropped my baby on his head. Would you mind picking her up while my accomplice checks out your back pocket?"* Or *"Pardon me for pouring that ketchup on your lovely sweater. Let me look in your purse for a hankie!"*) Scams can in fact be quite elaborate and you might not realize you are the victim of one until you go looking for your wallet, camera or iPod.
- Consider taking along your own padlock for your hotel room door.
- Don't open your room door unless you are absolutely sure who is on the other side.
- Learn the location of hotel exits and stairways in case you need to make a quick departure.
- Take along a flashlight and extra batteries.
- Don't walk alone in dark, isolated areas, or even in some of them if you have company. Romantic strolls on the beach are not always a good idea. Think twice in some well-lit areas as well.
- If you will be in a country for some time, or if there is significant unrest in that country, register with your local embassy or consulate. Make sure that someone you trust knows of your whereabouts at all times.
- Walk with some purpose in your step. That is, at least try to look like you know where you are going.
- Don't abuse alcohol. It may lead you into unsafe vehicles, unsafe sex and unsafe back alleys. An intoxicated tourist makes a much better target. The potency of local Russian vodka and Peruvian chicha may be greater than you think.

- Don't accept a drink from someone you don't know unless you saw it being poured.
- Avoid riots and political demonstrations, and generally stay away from unruly crowds. These websites will alert you to countries that are considered unsafe to visit — U.S. Department of State: http://travel.state.gov/travel_warnings.html; Canadian Department of Foreign Affairs and International Trade: www.voyage.gc.ca/consular_home-e.htm; www.voyage.gc.ca/countries_pays/menu-eng.asp
- Don't carry packages across borders for people you do not know, and even for some you do.

Remember that while you are away, you are subject to the laws of that country — not the land of your origin. If you are caught using or trafficking illegal drugs, or are suspected of any other crime, you may languish for years behind bars, which would prove hazardous to your health. Neither your high-priced lawyer back home nor your local government officials will wield much influence in such situations. Some offenses may be punishable by death.

Well if this list hasn't scared you to death, then you are ready to go! But please, use your common sense and be aware of your surroundings.

SEXUALLY TRANSMITTED INFECTIONS (STIs)

There is no shortage of statistics in the press regarding the prevalence of HIV in less developed countries. And there is no shortage of STIs above and beyond HIV, some of which are resistant to many antibiotics. Therefore, all travelers need to be very aware of the risks involved and the measures necessary to reduce these risks. Travelers do return infected with HIV and much more. The risk is real.

What about travelers?

While they may be well-informed, travelers are not always well behaved. The rate of casual sex is much higher than expected, and the use of condoms much lower. For some, sex is the sole purpose of their trip abroad, just as climbing Mount Kilimanjaro is for others. Commercial sexual exploitation of children is rampant around the world. While not all casual sex abroad could be described as "sexual tourism," exposure does occur among all groups, male and female, young and old, backpackers and businesspersons, and medical professionals and missionaries.

It is probably fair to say that inhibitions are lessened in many while abroad, perhaps because of the anonymity of travel. Isolation, the availability of sexual partners, alcohol and a desire to experience "something new" are other factors. To be fair, when I recently cautioned a patient about the risks of unprotected sex, he replied, *"Hell, I won't even touch the water!"*

Why is the situation different "over there"?

There are several reasons why the prevalence of STIs is greater in less developed countries:

1. HIV is transmitted primarily through heterosexual sex, putting many more people at risk.

2. Blood, blood products and medical instruments such as syringes are much more likely to be contaminated.
3. Infections causing genital ulcers are much more common, and these make the transmission of the HIV virus much more efficient.
4. Promiscuity and contact with prostitutes is extremely common.
5. Drugs that can reduce the transmission of HIV from pregnant mother to child may not be readily available or affordable in less developed countries.
6. Intravenous drug abuse is widespread in some countries.
7. Educational and public health measures have been unable to stem the epidemic in many places.

STIs are transmitted through unprotected sex. As well, infections such as HIV and hepatitis B and C can also be contracted through unsafe medical care, tattoos, acupuncture, and intravenous drug use. Thankfully mosquitoes, casual contact (hugging, kissing) and toilet seats are not responsible.

What are the symptoms of STIs?

The answer to this one will vary from person to person, and infection to infection. First, the incubation period (the time from exposure until the appearance of symptoms), varies greatly among these infections. Gonorrhea or chlamydia may produce symptoms in as few as three days, while infection with HIV or hepatitis B may not be detectable for two months or more. Women infected with gonorrhea or chlamydia often have no symptoms.

If you develop any of the following symptoms you must seek medical attention:

- discharge from the vagina or penis

- painful urination
- sores, ulcers or growths around the genitals or anus
- a rash
- swollen glands in the groin

These may only be the early or initial symptoms. While many sexually transmitted diseases are treatable and curable, some, such as HIV, genital herpes, genital warts and hepatitis B and C, may be with you for life. They may also pose a risk to future sexual partners and unborn children. Let's hope I have at least got your attention, and now, please read on.

REDUCING THE RISK OF STIs

1. Remain celibate — it's the only method that is 100 percent effective.
2. Be monogamous with someone whose HIV status you know.
3. Avoid high-risk sexual partners (commercial sex workers).
4. Always use a latex condom.
5. Beware of local doctors, dentists and their medical instruments. Find out where you can get safe medical care before you need it.
6. Avoid injections and blood transfusions unless absolutely necessary.
7. Carry your own first aid kit with sterile syringes and suture equipment.
8. Be sure that you are vaccinated against hepatitis B.
9. Avoid IV drugs, tattoos, acupuncture and body piercing.
10. Carry adequate medical insurance, so that if you need to return home for safe medical treatment you can afford it.
11. If you are at greater risk by virtue of your occupation

(e.g., doctor or nurse), wear latex gloves and be very careful.

A FEW WORDS ABOUT CONDOMS

While they are not perfect, they are your best protection if you plan to be sexually active while away. They must be used every time. Restrict yourself to the use of latex condoms. If you have a latex allergy, use polyurethane. For females, don't count on your male partner to provide the condom. Carry your own. Female condoms are available as well, but they are not quite as effective as the male condom in preventing pregnancy or STIs.

Condoms should be stored away from heat and light. One final note: Up to one-third of condoms manufactured overseas may not measure up to North America's rigid standards, so take along your own.

Lubricants and spermicides will further reduce the risk of HIV transmission. However, be sure these are water-based (e.g., K-Y Jelly), as oil-based lubricants such as Vaseline and baby oils may weaken latex condoms.

What if you think you have been exposed to HIV?

If you're working abroad as a health care worker and have accidentally sustained a needle-stick injury, or if you have been sexually assaulted by an unknown assailant, it would be reasonable to immediately seek **post-exposure prophylaxis (PEP).** This treatment to reduce the risk of HIV transmission consists of 28 days of antiretroviral medications, and is probably only of benefit within the first 72 hours after exposure. Obviously, every health center in the developing world will not have this sort of treatment available, but if you're at high risk by nature of your occupation, you should find out what to do before anything happens.

Assuming it's available, the exact treatment offered will depend upon factors such as the type of exposure, the severity of the exposure, and the likelihood that the source of exposure was HIV positive. So a drop of blood on your intact skin from someone who is known to be HIV negative would not warrant treatment. A deep puncture wound from a needle previously used on an HIV-positive individual would necessitate four weeks of treatment with multiple medications. If you have been exposed through unsafe sex, you should be examined and tested for other STIs as well.

The joy of sex and the joy of travel do not have to be mutually exclusive. But before you go, make sure you're fully aware of the risks involved, and how you can minimize them.

PART 2

WHILE YOU'RE AWAY

Chapter 4

BITES AND STINGS

INSECTS

Bzzzzzzzzzzz! Swat! Itch! Scratch! Sting! Ouch! There must be a zillion critters out there waiting to get a piece of you. Many are just a nuisance, while others transmit serious and occasionally fatal conditions. Let's first talk about insects and the many diseases they transmit.

How can I avoid insect bites?

- Minimize outdoor exposure between dusk and dawn when the *Anopheles* mosquito bites (may hamper your social life).
- If in a malarious area, sleep under a bed net (treated with permethrin) or in a room with sealed windows and a ceiling fan.
- Wear protective clothing such as long sleeves and long pants, depending on the ambient temperature. In southern Africa, where tick typhus is more prevalent, use repellents and cover yourself up (long

sleeves and long pants with your socks tucked into them). Inspect yourself for ticks. If you see one, pull it out gently with tweezers.

- Use insect repellents containing DEET or other effective ingredients during the day if concerned about dengue fever, and between dusk and dawn for malaria-carrying mosquitoes.
- Wear light-colored clothing, which is less likely to attract mosquitoes.
- Avoid perfumes, aftershaves and the like, which may attract mosquitoes.

Which repellent should I use?

There are many insect repellents to choose from. Some are "natural" and others are not so natural! Let's take a look.

DEET (N,N-diethyl-meta-toluamide) is the most effective, longest-lasting repellent. The duration of protection depends on the percentage concentration. 30–50% DEET will provide good protection, although perhaps not perfect, for four to six hours. Higher concentrations are no longer available in North America. Over the years, DEET has earned a bad and undeserved reputation. Yes, it may melt your upholstery, your sunglasses, watchband or iPod, but it is unlikely to affect your skin or your health.

Sensible precautions include:

- Keep it away from your eyes, mouth and hands.
- Wash it off when you return indoors.
- Keep it off of your iPod, sunglasses and synthetic materials.
- For small children, an adult should apply it sparingly, keeping it away from the child's hands, eyes and mouth, and wash it off when you come indoors.

According to the U.S. Environmental Protection Agency, DEET is approved for use on children with no age restriction.

Canadian guidelines recommend that DEET not be used in infants under 6 months. Health Canada's guidelines for the use of DEET are as follows:

Adults and children over 12 years	Use up to 30% DEET (good for 6 hours).
Children 2–12 years	Use up to 10% DEET (good for 3 hours), applied 3 times a day.
Children 6 months–2 years	Use up to 10% DEET, no more than once daily.
Infants under 6 months	Do not use DEET-containing insect repellents.

Combinations of repellent and sunscreens are not recommended. If there is a need for sunscreen as well, it should be applied first, followed 20 minutes later by the insect repellent. DEET is available in sprays, lotions and towelettes, and you can find it mixed with aloe to make it cosmetically pleasing. Controlled release preparations (e.g., Ultrathon®), which give you longer protection while maintaining a low concentration, are also available. Finally, DEET is considered safe in pregnancy.

Picaridin is a lesser-known repellent that has been used in Europe for more than a decade (available there as Autan Bayrepel®). Its efficacy is probably equal to DEET. It is odorless and will not eat away at your iPod!

Citronella is a popular "natural" repellent which can be applied to the skin, or burned as candles or coils. It probably doesn't protect you for much more than an hour, so frequent applications are necessary. It should not be used on small children.

Soybean oil, available as Bite Blocker®, is safe for small children and provides more than three hours of protection from mosquitoes, and even longer for blackflies.

Lemon eucalyptus products are probably the equivalent of 25% DEET, providing about four hours of protection. They are not recommended for children under the age of three.

Permethrin does not repel insects; rather, it works on contact, and "knocks down" its unsuspecting victims. It is nontoxic and can be applied to clothing, making it ideal for those tick-infested hikes in Kruger National Park in South Africa. More important, permethrin-treated bed nets can provide protection for between six months and five years. You should be sleeping under one if you are in a malarious area.

Insect-borne Diseases

Mosquitoes	Ticks	Mites	Flies
malaria	tick typhus	scrub typhus	onchocerciasis
dengue fever	Rocky Mountain spotted fever	chiggers	myiasis
yellow fever	tularaemia	scabies	sleeping sickness
West Nile virus	Lyme disease		loa loa
filariasis	babesiosis		leishmaniasis
chikungunya virus	erlichiosis		
Japanese encephalitis	tick-borne encephalitis		

Bugs	Fleas	Lice
Chagas disease	plague	louse-borne typhus
	tungiasis	louse-borne relapsing fever

SNAKES

I really don't like snakes or scorpions. I get frightened just researching them on the Internet. While an estimated 30,000 to 40,000 deaths occur worldwide each year from snakebites, I have yet to hear of it happening to a traveler. The odd scorpion, jellyfish or spider bite — well, maybe! You should be more worried about buses and motorbikes, but let's discuss these topics anyway. First, the snakes.

Some generalizations:

- The risk of snakebite to most travelers is very low.
- Snakes are not very aggressive creatures — they bite only when provoked.
- Only a small minority of snakes are dangerously venomous to humans.
- Not all bites from poisonous snakes result in significant envenomation.

About 700 of the world's 3,200 snake species are venomous. Snakes do not hear sounds as we hear them. Instead, they rely on vibrations through the ground, which are sensed through a delicate organ at the base of a snake's jaw. (Snake charmers may play charming music, but that snake is actually swaying to the movement and the tapping foot of the charmer.)

There are five main families of poisonous snakes. Their names and most prominent family members are:

- Viperidae: viper, adder, asp
- Elapidae: cobra, krait, mamba, coral snake, Australian poisonous snakes, sea snake
- Colubridae: boomslang, bird snake
- Hydrophiidae: sea snake, sea krait

- Crotalidae (pit vipers): rattlesnake, American and Asian lancehead, copperhead, cottonmouth, fer-de-lance, bushmaster

All snakebites, regardless of their type, will probably cause immediate fright, which is understandable. The fright may cause the victim to quickly appear as if in shock; that is, semi-conscious, with cold, clammy skin, a feeble pulse and rapid, shallow breathing. This occurs much more quickly than the effects of any venom. Further symptoms depend on the type of venom and the severity of the bite, and may be divided into local and systemic effects.

Local effects — At the site of a poisonous bite, one may see two small holes, left there by the fangs of the snake. If the victim has had a nonpoisonous bite, the local reaction will be no worse than from any other bite. If venom has been injected, there will be immediate swelling, pain and discoloration of the surrounding skin. This is most typical of cobra and pit viper bites. These effects may proceed on to necrosis or death of the superficial tissues.

Systemic effects — Elapidae produce primarily a neurotoxin. Reactions include pain and muscular weakness. As well, the ability to swallow, speak, keep one's eyes open or breathe may be affected. Some cobras are able to project their venom several feet into the victim's eyes, causing intense pain and swelling. Sea snakes may cause the breakdown of the muscles (myotoxicity), neurotoxicity (damage to the nervous system) and kidney failure. Although death may occur as early as 15 minutes after an elapid bite, this is the exception and not the rule. As is the case with dog bites, there is usually time to get to qualified medical care.

Viperidae secrete a hemorrhagic toxin, which may be manifested by minor bleeding from the gums, or more serious bleeding into the internal organs (e.g., the intestines or brain). Shock may result from massive bleeding.

Some tips for avoiding snakes:

- Don't walk in unknown areas without footwear.
- Stay on the beaten path, especially at night.
- Beware of outhouses and latrines.
- Carry a flashlight and walking stick at night.
- Keep your hands away from rocks, woodpiles and holes in the ground.
- Don't swim in swamps or rivers matted with vegetation.
- Check under your clothing before getting dressed.
- If you encounter a snake, stay still (snakes prefer moving targets) until it slinks away.
- Keep a safe distance from snake charmers.

I got bitten. What should I do now?

- Do not panic!
- Remain calm and get the victim away from the snake.
- Do not attempt to catch and kill the snake. Even a severed head can bite.
- Immobilize the limb with a splint and keep it at or below the level of the heart.
- Call for help.
- Gently cleanse the wound to remove any excess venom. Do not apply ice, heat or a tourniquet to the wound. Do not administer aspirin.
- Remove rings, bracelets and other potentially con-stricting items.
- Apply a crepe bandage to the whole limb. The idea of this bandage is to slow venous and lymphatic flow. It

should not block the arterial blood flow. Make sure you can feel a pulse distal to the bandage (toward the extremities). Do not remove this bandage until you reach medical care and, if it's necessary, antivenin is at hand.

- If the snake is dead, take it to the hospital (on a stick). Otherwise, do your best to identify the snake.

When you have reached medical care, you will be monitored for signs of envenomation, such as bleeding, swelling or paralysis. If these appear, you should be treated with the appropriate antivenin. This is usually administered intravenously and very slowly. Allergic reactions to antivenin sometimes occur, so medical personnel must be prepared for that complication. Other treatments may include supportive care and antibiotics. Remember, snakebites are rare among travelers.

SCORPIONS

Scorpions are equipped with a pair of pincers used to hold on to prey, and a stinger. These arachnids tend to be nocturnal and are more active in hot, humid weather. Scorpions have their own outdoor hiding places, such as under rocks, wood and leaves, as well as indoor spots — in corners, inside shoes and under clothing. So shake out your sleeping bag, and check your tent before getting too comfortable, and check inside your shoes in the morning.

As with snakes, not all scorpion stings produce severe reactions. But when they do, children, by virtue of their smaller size, are at greatest risk. Intense pain may occur at the site of the sting, and this feeling may be associated with severe thirst, vomiting and diarrhea. The scorpion's venom has a neurotoxic effect and may cause respiratory paralysis or convulsions. Cardiovascular effects and hemorrhage may also occur. An acute anaphylactic (allergic) reaction may happen as well, requiring immediate treatment.

Anaphylaxis is, hopefully, treated with adrenaline (e.g., EpiPen®) and an antihistamine. Local pain can be controlled with topical cool compresses and potent painkillers. Antivenins may be available, but their use is a bit controversial. Once again, try to seek qualified medical care as quickly as possible.

SPIDERS

The most famous and dangerous spiders include the brown recluse spider, the black widow spider, the funnel web spider of Australia and tarantulas. Most of these spiders are not aggressive, so the trick is to keep your distance. They hang out in all the same places as scorpions.

Spider bites usually cause local pain, redness and swelling. But tissue damage and muscle spasm, progressing to nerve dysfunction and respiratory difficulty, may occur. Treatment consists of immobilization of the affected extremity and compression with a bandage and ice. Analgesics and antivenin should be given if necessary.

Centipedes, fire ants, beetles and many more creepy crawlers are out there, but in general, you are not part of their usual diet. Try to keep out of their way, and they may keep out of yours.

SOME OTHER CREATURES

Jellyfish, and a few of their relatives, belong to the family known as coelenterates. They transmit their toxins to us by means of an ingenious mechanism called a nematocyst. There are millions of these on the tentacles of the jellyfish. On contact with living tissue (you or me), small tubes in the nematocyst puncture your skin and inject their poison directly into your small blood vessels.

The species responsible for the most deaths worldwide are the chirodropids, commonly called box jellyfish, which are found mainly off the shores of North Queensland, Australia and in Southeast Asia. Their sting can cause death from cardiac arrest within 60 seconds. They get washed onto shore by the currents, wind and tides, and are usually not easy to see. Thus, the symptoms are usually a bit unexpected.

The initial symptom of a jellyfish sting is intense pain at the site of the "bite." Rapid death from severe envenomation can also be one of the initial symptoms. The skin may be red, discolored or blistered, and the linear pattern of the tentacles can usually be seen. It may look as if you were branded. Women and children are more susceptible to severe stings, perhaps because of their relatively hairless legs. Most stings occur on the lower legs, until you start to pick at the tentacles, at which point they also occur on the hands and arms. Other symptoms of envenomation may include nausea and vomiting, pains in the joints, wheezing and difficulty breathing, and paralysis.

To treat jellyfish stings:

- Prevent drowning and remove the victim from the scene.
- Pour on five percent acetic acid, better known as vinegar. This solution will inactivate the nematocyst

toxins. Rubbing alcohol or urine, also effective, may be more immediately available.

- Wash off any remaining tentacles with seawater. Fresh water or hot water will cause the remaining nematocysts to fire.
- Gently remove remaining nematocysts with shaving cream and a razor, not with vigorous rubbing.
- Provide pain relief, topical ice packs and other supportive measures (e.g., oxygen and intravenous fluids).
- Control the pain and prevent further absorption of poison by using compression bandages and immobilization.
- Make sure the victim is given tetanus toxoid if necessary. In Australia, antivenin is available for severe envenomation from box jellyfish.

The **Portuguese man-of-war** (*Physalia physalis*) is found along both the Atlantic and Pacific coasts. This creature can cause extremely painful stings, although death is uncommon. Tentacles that have washed up on the beach and may look "dead" are still capable of envenomation.

Sea urchins are a bit like aquatic porcupines. When we accidentally step on them or handle them, their spines penetrate our skin and may cause severe, burning pain along with local swelling, redness and muscle aches. Generalized symptoms such as nausea and vomiting, muscle weakness and low blood pressure may occur with multiple puncture wounds. This time, hot water for about an hour (not urine or seawater) is the best treatment. Spines that may have broken off in the skin should be removed if possible, as they may go on to cause chronic problems if left in place. These wounds often become infected, so preventive antibiotics are a good idea.

Starfish are also covered with spines that may be venomous.

Fortunately, there is only one important poisonous starfish, which is located in the Pacific. *Acanthaster planci*, commonly known as the crown-of-thorns starfish, causes immediate pain, redness and swelling when touched. Other symptoms may include numbness, nausea, vomiting and muscle weakness. If possible, broken spines should be removed. Hot water is the treatment of choice.

Sea cucumbers are bottom feeders that also possess nematocysts. Contact with the tentacles usually causes only a mild skin irritation, but if you touch your eyes severe inflammation may occur. Treat this inflammation with topical anesthetics, irrigation (of your eye) and a quick visit to an eye doctor.

Coral tends to attract divers like a magnet. It is actually a living creature, and some species may have nematocysts. The main complication of cuts from coral is secondary bacterial infection. Treatment consists of thorough cleansing with soap and water or other antiseptics, as well as topical and oral antibiotics. If stinging is present, vinegar or urine will deactivate the firing nematocysts.

Fire coral, which actually looks like true coral, attaches itself to rocks and coral. Divers who lean against or handle coral are often in for a painful surprise.

Now, let's finish with something completely different …

The **candiru fish** (*Vandellia cirrhosa*) is a delightful parasitic catfish that is found in the waters of the Amazon and Orinoco Rivers of South America. It's a bit of a vampire, and its main target is the gills of other fish, where it anchors itself and feeds on their blood.

If you are swimming in the buff and happen to heed nature's call to empty your bladder, this little guy (about an inch long) will be attracted to you. After having found the source of the urine, he will then swim upstream into your urethra, lodge itself with its spines and gorge itself on your blood. This is, in fact, a big mistake for the fish, since once he is engorged and stuck, there is no way out. It's also bad news for you, because the pain, I am told, is something else. There are treatments available, but avoidance is the best policy!

So what have we learned? Cover up, use your insect repellent and know when to pee and when not to.

Chapter 5

MALARIA

Malaria is the greatest infectious threat to travelers going to the tropics. It is also one of the greatest threats to children living in the tropics. More than one million children die from malaria every year in SubSaharan Africa. The main reason is poverty. Treated bed nets may be unaffordable. Medical care or treatment may be inadequate, too expensive or unavailable. Education regarding the treatment of fever may be lacking. And finally, an effective vaccine, which has been on the horizon for years, is still not available.

For the traveler, it should be a preventable infection and, if necessary, a treatable one. You will hear lots of information about malaria and antimalarials before you go and while you are away. Much of it will be misleading or downright dangerous. What follows is the truth.

What is malaria?

Malaria is a parasitic (protozoan, to be more specific) infection of the red blood cells that is transmitted by the bite of the female *Anopheles* mosquito. There are four human strains of this parasite: *Plasmodium vivax*, *Plasmodium ovale*, *Plasmodium malariae* and *Plasmodium falciparum*. Of the four, it is this last strain, *P. falciparum*, that has developed resistance to many antimalarial drugs. It also happens to be the only strain that may prove fatal (there may be exceptions with *P. vivax* in Papua New Guinea). *P. vivax* and *P. ovale* have the ability to lie dormant in the liver for longer periods, and hence may account for cases of malaria that occur months after exposure, or cases that relapse. *P. malariae* is the least commonly encountered strain. A monkey strain of malaria, *P. knowlesii*, has recently been discovered in humans as well.

After being injected into your bloodstream, the young parasites, or sporozoites, quickly find their way to your liver. Here they spend a minimum of six days dividing, though they can sometimes remain dormant for weeks and months (hypnozoites). From there they travel to your bloodstream and invade the red blood cells (trophozoites). Once again, they start to divide (schizonts), and after 24 to 72 hours they finally turn into between 8 and 24 new parasites (merozoites). The red blood cells eventually rupture, releasing these new, young parasites to invade even more red blood cells.

After a few of these cycles, more and more red blood cells become infected and you become sicker and sicker. With *P. falciparum*, this may lead to **cerebral malaria**, not a strain of malaria but a dreaded complication that often proves fatal. As well, some of the parasites develop into gametocytes, the sexual form, and are picked up by the next feeding mosquito before being passed on to someone else.

What are the symptoms?

The symptoms of malaria are legion. It can mimic almost any other disease, but I would suggest you concentrate on the following:

- fever (measured by a thermometer)

- headache
- chills and the shakes
- aches and pains
- fatigue
- feeling extremely cold, followed by the opposite, and then, a drenching sweat

These symptoms may in fact disappear, only to return in 48 to 72 hours, as the dividing parasites become "synchronized." Should the infection go untreated, more red blood cells become destroyed, and you become anemic. In the case of *P. falciparum*, cerebral malaria, which is characterized by headache, confusion, seizures or coma may occur and can cause death in as little as three days from the onset of the fever. The lungs and kidneys can also be seriously affected.

There are many other causes of fever and headache when you are in the tropics. Dengue fever, typhoid fever, tick typhus, meningitis, leptospirosis, hepatitis and Lassa fever are just a few. Don't forget that "Western" illnesses such as kidney infections, influenza, pneumonia or mononucleosis can also occur.

How do you get it?

That's fairly simple. As mentioned, malaria is transmitted through the bite of the female *Anopheles* mosquito. She requires human blood for the development of her young. This strain of mosquito prefers to breed in stagnant bodies of water, and the females do their biting between dusk and dawn. What do male mosquitoes do in their evenings, you may ask? Drink, sleep or watch NFL football are some of the suggestions I have heard. Malaria can also be passed on from pregnant mother to baby at birth, and through blood transfusions, which is why The Red Cross will decline your blood donation for at least a year after you have visited a malarious area. Consider donating before you travel.

Where do you get it?

The maps on the following pages give you an idea of where there is risk of malaria. But such maps can overstate the risk. Let me give you a few generalizations with respect to the distribution of malaria.

Caribbean and Central America — limited to Haiti, most of the Dominican Republic and lowland rural (not urban) areas in Central America.

South America — mainly in the Amazon Basin; not in urban areas or at high altitudes.

Asia (India, Pakistan, Bangladesh) — present in urban and rural areas; may be seasonal depending on the temperature and rainfall; not at high altitudes.

Southeast Asia and China — mainly in rural areas, not urban areas or coastal resorts; in China, only in rural areas in the south.

Africa — in sub-Saharan Africa, present in urban and rural areas, with a few exceptions such as the cities of Nairobi and Addis Ababa; in South Africa, mainly in the northeast Transvaal, or Kruger National Park.

Oceania — islands such as Papua New Guinea, Vanuatu and the Solomon Islands have a high risk of malaria.

As far as the relative risk of acquiring malaria, it is highest in Oceania and sub-Saharan Africa; moderate in Asia; and lowest in Southeast Asia, Central America and South America. So, if your plans are to vagabond through the Andes from Ecuador to Bolivia, but not soak your feet in the Amazon, you will not need antimalarials. If your idea of traveling through Southeast Asia means visiting Bangkok,

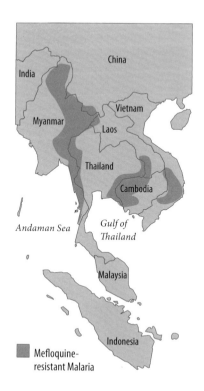

China

India

Vietnam

Myanmar

Laos

Thailand

Cambodia

Andaman Sea

Gulf of Thailand

Malaysia

Indonesia

Mefloquine-resistant Malaria

Chang Mai, Singapore, Kuala Lumpur, Hong Kong and Bali, the same applies. If it is Cairo to Capetown, you won't need antimalarials in those two cities — but you will everywhere in between.

In some places, malaria may be a seasonal risk. New Delhi or Kruger National Park in their respective winters might harbor little or no risk. The best place to look up the risk at your destination is the Centers for Disease Control and Prevention (CDC) website (www.cdc.gov/MALARIA/risk_map/), where you can dial up your country. As well, a travel medicine specialist should be well acquainted with the distribution of malaria.

Countries Reporting Cases of Malaria

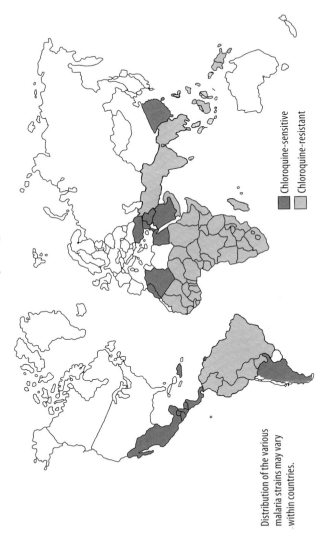

Chloroquine-sensitive

Chloroquine-resistant

Distribution of the various malaria strains may vary within countries.

Malaria

How do you prevent it?

By taking personal protective measures and taking the proper antimalarials properly, malaria should be totally preventable. But as mentioned, not everyone takes these precautions, either because of misinformation or, I suppose, personal preference.

PERSONAL PROTECTIVE MEASURES

- Minimize outdoor exposure between dusk and dawn.
- Wear light-colored clothing.
- Wear long sleeves and pants.
- Avoid perfumes and aftershaves, as they may attract mosquitoes.
- Sleep in a well-screened, air-conditioned room.
- Use an insect repellent containing DEET, or another effective alternative. (See Chapter 4.)
- Sleep under a treated bed net (treated with permethrin).

ANTIMALARIAL MEDICATIONS

The ideal antimalarial would be 100 percent effective, free of side effects, convenient to take, safe in pregnancy and inexpensive. The ones we have probably provide about 95 percent protection. We don't really have a perfect antimalarial, but almost everyone should be able to tolerate one of the following options. The antimalarial you choose depends on the following:

- Your destination. Is there malaria in the area? Is it chloroquine-sensitive malaria?
- Your personal medical history. Are you pregnant? Have you suffered from depression? Do you have epilepsy? Do you have any allergies?

- Your age.
- Your budget. One of the antimalarials, Malarone®, can be exceedingly expensive, especially if you are exposed for a long time.
- Your past experience with antimalarials and your personal preference.

CHLOROQUINE (NIVAQUINE®, ARALEN®)

There was a time when chloroquine was adequate to prevent and treat all forms of malaria. But since the Vietnam War in the 1960s it's been losing its efficacy, and now would be effective only in parts of Mexico, Central America, Haiti, the Dominican Republic and the Middle East. It is convenient, being taken on a weekly basis, starting the week before your trip, each week you are exposed, and for four weeks after you leave the malarious area. Side effects include an upset stomach, headache and, in those with black skin, itchiness. The taste is bitter — to say the least — so it should be taken quickly with lots of food and water. For children, it could be crushed up and mixed with something pleasant. It should be avoided by anyone with psoriasis or epilepsy. Chloroquine is safe in pregnancy and is inexpensive. It can be quite toxic if taken in excess, so keep the bottle away from children. If taken for a prolonged time (several years), there is risk of damage to the retina, so yearly eye exams would be recommended.

MEFLOQUINE (LARIAM®)

This drug has aroused more controversy than most since it was introduced in the 1960s, mainly because of its actual or alleged side effects. But it continues to be a useful antimalarial because of its convenience and low cost. It is effective against chloroquine-resistant malaria everywhere, with the exception of along the Thai-Cambodian and Thai-Burmese borders.

Mefloquine is taken on a weekly basis, ideally beginning about three weeks prior to departure (to catch side effects before you actually leave); weekly while exposed; and for four weeks after leaving the malarious area. It needs to be taken on a full stomach with lots of water, and it should not be taken on the same day as alcohol. Taking it in the morning or the evening may or may not affect your side effects.

Mefloquine should be avoided in people with a history of the following:

- anxiety, depression or psychosis (past or present)
- epilepsy
- disorders of cardiac conduction (irregular heart rhythms)
- intolerable side effects in the past

Its most common side effects, which may occur in about 15 percent of people, include:

- vivid dreams — they may be erotic, exotic or scary and you may feel like you were awake during the dream
- dizziness, insomnia, upset stomach
- mood changes such as anxiety or depression

It is this last side effect that may be most distressing, and it would certainly be reason enough to stop the mefloquine and consider an alternative. Young women are probably the most susceptible to this effect, and children are rarely affected. Side effects may be transient and tolerable (mefloquine Mondays) and may be minimized by taking one-half pill twice weekly. Much rarer side effects include seizures and psychosis. Mefloquine is considered safe in the second and third trimester of pregnancy, and would probably be the best choice if first trimester travel was unavoidable.

DOXYCYCLINE (VIBRAMYCIN®)

This antibiotic is effective against all strains of malaria. It is taken on a daily basis, beginning one or two days before exposure, daily while away and for 28 days after leaving the malarious area. It must be taken with food and lots of water during the day while you are upright. There are three main side effects to be aware of:

- Photosensitivity — so sunscreens and protective clothing are a must, especially for the fair and sensitive.
- Predisposition to vaginal yeast infections or oral thrush — so carry along some curative treatment such as Monistat® or Diflucan®.
- Heartburn or esophagitis may occur, hence the need to take it as instructed.

Doxycycline can cause a yellow staining of the developing teeth, so it must not be used in children under eight, or in pregnant or nursing mothers.

MALARONE® (ATOVAQUONE/PROGUANIL)

This medication, actually a combination of medications, has been used since the start of the 21st century, and it gives excellent protection against all forms of malaria. It is taken daily, starting the day before exposure, daily while away, and for only seven days after leaving the malarious area. Its side effects are relatively uncommon, but they may include gastro-intestinal upset and mouth ulcers (especially in kids wearing braces). It is not recommended in pregnancy. Due to its high cost of about $5 CDN a pill, it is not affordable to everyone, but it will be attractive for shorter-term travelers as well as those with drug insurance or lots of money. It is available in pediatric strengths.

PRIMAQUINE

This is an older medication which has traditionally been used to eradicate the persistent forms of malaria in the liver (*P. vivax* and *P. ovale*), but which has been found to be very effective in preventing all strains of malaria. It is taken on a daily basis, starting the day before exposure, daily while away and for only seven days after leaving the malarious area. Before taking primaquine, you must have a blood test to ensure that you have an adequate level of the enzyme G6PD. It is not recommended in pregnancy.

What if I get malaria (or think I have it)?

If you are traveling in malarious areas, the chances of being diagnosed with malaria are probably greater than your actually having it. This applies especially if you are taking your antimalarials properly. Experience tells me that you should be prepared for both scenarios: being diagnosed, and catching malaria. In addition, malaria often doesn't strike until you have returned home, so in that case, you and your doctor must follow the rule: *"Fever in a returning traveler is malaria until proven otherwise."*

The diagnosis of malaria is made by observing the parasites in a blood smear. This test requires time, technology and training, and it may not be the procedure in the proverbial middle of nowhere. Other automated tests, such as MalaQuick®, OptiMAL®, ICT Malaria Pf® and ParaSight-F®, are a little simpler and, in trained hands, highly accurate. These are known as RDTs (rapid diagnostic tests).

Studies in travelers have shown that malaria is undoubtedly overdiagnosed in the tropics (See Medical Care Abroad in Chapter 1). Although unneeded treatment may not pose a great risk to the patient, it can be a concern for a few reasons. First, the correct diagnosis may be delayed. Second, when even mild illness is treated as malaria, people will begin to believe that malaria is a mild illness, which it isn't. Finally, many individuals will discontinue their antimalarials and tell others that they were ineffective.

But back home, **malaria runs the dangerous risk of being under-diagnosed**. Doctors are not on the watch for tropical infections unless you tell them you have recently returned from the tropics. Keep in mind, no matter where your fever turns up, that a negative test for malaria does not necessarily mean you don't have malaria. If your fever persists without any other obvious cause, you should return to the doctor to repeat the test until a diagnosis is made or your fever disappears.

Artemisinin and its derivatives, used in the treatment of uncomplicated malaria, have been available in the tropics for several years. There they are available as pills, injections and suppositories. Coartem® (artemether/lumefantrine) has recently become available in North America for treatment. It is hoped that by using a combination therapy, drug resistance will be delayed or prevented.

Complicated malaria, say when more than five percent of the red blood cells contain parasites, requires expert and intensive treatment. Remember, malaria is a treatable and curable infection if treated promptly and properly.

MALARIA MYTHS

There are probably more myths and misconceptions about malaria than about most diseases. Permit me to dispel most of them. (The myths are in italic, the truth in regular type.)

1. *Taking antimalarials only masks the disease.* Chloroquine, mefloquine and doxycycline kill the malaria parasites in the bloodstream. Malarone® and primaquine do so in the liver. So while none of them actually prevents infection, they do prevent the symptoms of the disease, including death.

2. *If I take antimalarials, there will be nothing left to treat me*

with if I get sick. While extra caution may be needed when using certain drugs together, this certainly does not preclude effective treatment.

3. *If I am taking antimalarials, it will make it more difficult for the doctors to diagnose it if I get infected*. Not correct. First, you probably won't get malaria. Second, if there are malaria parasites there, they should be visible under the microscope. This may take a good lab technician and more than one blood smear, but if the parasites are truly there, they should be seen.

4. *The drugs are worse than the disease*. Again, any of the aforementioned side effects of any of the medications do not compare with the discomfort and possible fatal outcome of having malaria.

5. *I am immune to malaria*. Those who grew up in malarious areas such as Africa may indeed have developed some relative immunity to this infection. However, this protection tends to wane with time, and cannot be counted on for that next trip back home.

6. *Once you have malaria, you have it for life*. Not true. While I have seen numerous patients who are convinced that they have suffered relapses on a yearly basis since World War II, this is rarely the case. As I mentioned, there are two strains, *P. vivax* and *P. ovale*, which may persist for months and even years in your liver, but they can easily be eradicated with the drug primaquine.

7. *You must not take antimalarials for an extended period of time*. Not true. If you feel well on your antimalarial, you may continue it indefinitely (remember, long-term use of chloroquine necessitates a regular eye check). Some European countries establish limits on antimalarial drugs, but in North America we do not.

Summary of Antimalarials

Medication	Adult dosage	How to take it	Pediatric dosage	Comments
chloroquine (Aralen®, Nivaquine®)	1 tablet = 150 mg base = 250 mg salt	Take 2 tablets weekly beginning 1 week prior to exsorsure, weekly while away and for 4 weeks after your return.	5 mg/kg base weekly to maximum 300 mg or 1–2 yrs: 75 mg base 3–4 yrs: 100 mg base 5–7 yrs: 125 mg base 8–10 yrs: 200 mg base 11–13 yrs: 250 mg base > 14 yrs: 300 mg base	• tastes bitter; may be crushed up and mixed with food • toxic if taken in overdose • available as a liquid overseas • safe in pregnancy
mefloquine (Lariam®)	250 mg tablets	Take 1 tablet weely, beginning 1 week prior to travel, weekly while away and for 4 weeks after your return.	< 15 kg: 5 mg/kg/wk 15–19 kg: ¼ tablet/wk 20–30 kg: ½ tablet/wk 31–45 kg: ¾ tablet/wk > 45 kg: 1 tablet/wk	• take with food and lots of water, not alcohol • contraindicated with epilepsy, psychiatric disorders, cardiac conduction disturbances
doxycycline (Vibramycin®)	100 mg tablets	Take 1 tablet daily, beginning the day before exposure, daily while away and for weeks after your return.	> 8 yrs: 2 mg/kg of body weight once/day, up to the adult dose of 100 mg	• contraindicated during pregnancy and breastfeeding, and under the age of 8 • take with food and lots of water during the day
atovaquone/ proguanil (Malarone®)	250 mg tablets/100 mg tablets	Take 1 tablet daily, beginning the day before exposure, daily while exposed and for 7 days after your return.	11–20 kg: 62.5/25 mg 21–30 kg: 125/50 mg 31–40 kg: 187.5/75 mg > 40 kg: 250/100 mg (1 tablet)	• contraindicated in pregnancy • commonest side effects are gastrointestinal and mouth ulcers
primaquine	15 mg tablets (base)	Take 2 tablets (30 mg) daily, beginning the day before exposure, daily while away and for 7 days after your return.	0.5 mg/kg base daily to maximum 30 mg/day	• must check G6PD level prior to taking it • contraindicated in pregnancy

Note: Check dosages and instructions with doctor or pharmacist.

131

PART 3

AFTER YOU'RE BACK

Now that your bags are unpacked, you've sorted out your 20,000 digital photos and your laundry is done, the question comes up, "Do I need to see a doctor?" That depends. There are four kinds of returning travelers:

1. Those who weren't at great risk, who feel great when they get home and stay that way.
2. Those who feel great when they get home but develop illness after their arrival home.
3. Those who get off the plane with a fever of 39°C/101°F and dreadful diarrhea.
4. Those who feel great, but were at higher risk and may have been exposed to infections such as HIV, TB, schistosomiasis, intestinal worms, etc.

Those in the first group really don't need to see the doctor. They had a lovely week or two on safari and can now plan their next trip. But let's talk about the others and some of the problems they may have. Remember that all of these problems may also occur while you are still away.

It wouldn't hurt to have a checkup when you get home, particularly if you have been away for some time and possibly exposed to many infections. Hopefully, the doctor will ask you some of the same old questions such as:

- Where have you been?
- When and for how long were you there?
- What were you doing over there?
- Did you have any illnesses while away?
- Did you swim in fresh water, walk barefoot, have unprotected sex or unsafe injections?

Then, after a thorough physical exam, some routine tests may be advisable, depending upon your answers to the above. These tests might include:

- CBC (complete blood count)
- stools for ova and parasites (O & P)
- serology – testing for antibodies to certain infections such as schistosomiasis, filariasis, etc.
- TB skin test – this should be done about two months after your return. If it is positive, and was negative before you left, then you have developed a "latent" infection with tuberculosis. You are not contagious or ill, but run the risk of developing "active" TB down the road. The risk of this happening is greatest in the first two years after your return. To minimize this risk, the doctor may recommend a course of the drug INH (isoniazid) for 6 to 12 months.
- HIV, VDRL, cervical or urethral swabs if you may have been exposed to STIs or unsafe injections

Most travelers who return well, are well. But don't forget the possibility that malaria might surface weeks and months after your return. Fatigue is another common problem in returning travelers. Possible causes may include jet lag, reverse culture shock and depression, various infections or perhaps some post-travel variant of chronic fatigue syndrome.

This chapter does not mention every "tropical" disease known, but it does cover the most common problems that occur in returning travelers. Hopefully, you have returned with none of the above. But even if you have, don't let that discourage you from planning your next adventure. Worms go away, but the memories last forever!

Chapter 6

WELCOME HOME

Fever in a returning traveler is malaria until proven otherwise. If both you and your doctor follow this dictum, you should be OK. The most serious strain, *P. falciparum*, will usually cause symptoms within 60 days of your return. The other more benign strains may in fact rest in your liver for months before making you sick. Malaria is usually accompanied by other symptoms such as:

- headache
- chills and the shakes
- body aches and pains
- feeling very hot, and then very cold
- weakness and fatigue
- and don't forget the fever!

Malaria can mimic almost any illness. If it goes untreated, *P. falciparum* may progress to cerebral malaria (confusion, seizures, coma and death) or respiratory failure in as little as three days. The bottom line: if you have a fever on your return, see a doctor — a doctor who knows something about malaria.

There are several other infections that may cause fever upon your return. God only gave us a limited number of symptoms, so things can get a bit confusing! They are listed in the table below.

Common Causes of Tropical Fevers in Returning Travelers	
malaria	tick typhus
typhoid fever	leptospirosis
hepatitis A	*Shigella*
Salmonella	*Campylobacter*
dengue fever	malaria (just a reminder!)

Most of the clues to your illness lie your recent medical history.

- **Where were you?** Were you actually in a malarious area or an area with an outbreak of dengue? Or perhaps in West Africa with Lassa fever?
- **When were you there?** The incubation period, that is, the time from when you were exposed to the time when you became ill, is extremely important. If you develop your fever three weeks after your return, you don't have dengue, but you may have malaria, typhoid fever or hepatitis A.
- **What vaccines did you receive before you left?** If you were immunized against hepatitis A and B and yellow fever, it is highly unlikely that you are ill with these infections. Remember, typhoid vaccine is only about 65 percent effective.
- **Are you taking/did you take your antimalarials properly?** This is not a guarantee that you can't get malaria, but it makes malaria less likely.

- **What other exposures did you have?** Visiting game parks in southern Africa might suggest tick typhus. Rafting in polluted waters might result in leptospirosis. Receiving questionable injections might lead to hepatitis B, C or HIV.
- **What other symptoms and signs do you have?** Do you have a rash? (dengue, meningococcal disease); Is there an ulcer or eschar on your leg? (tick typhus); Are you turning yellow? (hepatitis); Do you have bloody diarrhea? (*Campylobacter*, *Shigella*, *Salmonella*, amebiasis)

Obviously, North American diseases such as influenza, pneumonia, strep throat, infectious mononucleosis, kidney infection, etc., can also occur when you return to North America. Make sure the doctor knows that you have been away though. He or she might not ask!

The investigation of the returned traveler with a fever may include any or all of the following:

- complete blood count — might give a clue to what you have
- malaria smear or an "automated" test for malaria
- urinalysis
- tests of liver function
- blood, urine, stool cultures
- chest x-ray
- abdominal ultrasound
- serological tests — checking for antibodies
- anything else, depending upon your history and physical findings

One important rule:

If your malaria smear was negative, that doesn't mean you

don't have malaria. It means they didn't find it the first time. This test should be repeated again and again as long as you continue to have fever or until another diagnosis is made.

Patients have died because this rule was not followed. In up to a third of cases, a cause for the fever may not be found and the patient will recover.

Obviously the treatment of your illness will depend upon the diagnosis. Were you to develop the same problem in Africa, the doctor would probably treat you right off the bat with antimalarials for malaria and antibiotics for typhoid and everything else. That might in fact be a successful strategy. Back home, your doctor is more likely to wait for the actual diagnosis.

Just a word about the treatment of malaria, which should probably be undertaken under the supervision of a tropical or infectious disease specialist. The treatment will depend upon the strain of malaria that you have, the medications that are available and how sick you are.

Chloroquine-sensitive malaria — can be treated with chloroquine over three days; if you have *P. vivax* or *P. ovale*, which can persist in your liver, then you need a 14-day course of primaquine. Before taking this drug, you must ensure that you have a normal G6PD level.

Chloroquine-resistant malaria — (usually *P. falciparum*) in the patient who is not that ill and can be relied upon to take the medication, there are a few choices:

- Oral quinine for seven days along with another medication such as doxycycline (not very pleasant).
- Malarone® four tablets per day for three days.
- Artemesinin-combined therapy (ACT) that consists of artemesinin in combination with another antimalarial. Coartem®/Riamet® (artemether/

139

lumenfantrine) taken for three days is highly effective and has recently become available in North America.

- More serious or complicated cases of malaria (cerebral malaria, severe anemia or lung involvement) will need to be treated in hospital with intensive therapy.

Remember, fever in a returning traveler is malaria until proven otherwise. Malaria is a very treatable infection if treated promptly and properly. Get to the doctor quickly, and mention that you were in Gabon, India, Indonesia, Peru or anywhere else!

STOMACH TROUBLES

Gastrointestinal problems, especially diarrhea, are the commonest ailments in returning travelers. Many will have this on or within a few days of their return. Others may take a few weeks to develop symptoms and the symptoms may drag on. There are a host of things that might have hitched a free ride home to North America by way of your intestines. Your doctor might ask you the following questions:

- **Where have you been and how careful were you?** While you can pick up almost anything almost anywhere, certain infections are more likely in certain locales and under certain conditions.
- **When did you return?** Again, incubation periods are important. Bacterial infections (*E. coli, Salmonella, Shigella, Campylobacter*) usually have a brief incubation period of only a few days. Parasites (giardiasis, amebiasis, *Cyclospora, Cryptosporidium*) may take longer to strike.
- **What other symptoms do you have?** Fever and blood or mucus in your stools (dysentery) suggests a more "invasive" infection, such as a bacterial type or perhaps amebiasis. Gas, bloating, rumbling, farts that curl your nose, and lactose intolerance are characteristic of giardiasis or other intestinal amebas. Remember that if you have a fever, malaria needs to be considered as well.

The initial investigation of the returned traveler with diarrhea starts with:

- stool culture (C & S) — to grow bacteria
- stool for ova and parasites (O & P) — to find intestinal parasites (worms and protozoa) and to look for

white and red blood cells suggestive of dysentery. Some intestinal amebas are "non-pathogenic," that is, unlikely to make you very sick.

The above two tests involve getting a small amount of stool into a very small bottle. I will leave the "how" to you! Other tests, depending upon the initial results, will depend upon the history and the course of the patient's illness. That is, if the traveler is all better, it probably won't be necessary to do any more tests. If further tests are required, they may include:

- complete blood count
- tests of intestinal absorption — iron, folic acid levels and lactose tolerance test
- thyroid function — an overactive thyroid can cause diarrhea
- serological tests — antibodies to *Entameba histolytica* (amebiasis)
- gastroscopy — looking for causes of malabsorption such as celiac disease, tropical sprue, giardiasis and *H. pylori* (not a cause of diarrhea but rather "ulcer-like" pain)
- colonoscopy — looking for inflammatory bowel disease, invasive amebiasis or cancer

Again, remember that not everything that happens after returning from the tropics is "tropical." Inflammatory bowel disease (ulcerative colitis, Crohn's disease), lactose intolerance, hyperthyroidism, cancer of the bowel or ovary, celiac disease and much more can affect your bowels.

Perhaps the commonest diagnosis you are left with after a full investigation is a post-infectious irritable bowel syndrome. This means: *"I spent two years in [insert the name of your country here]. I got sick several times. I got better. But I'm still not the way I was before."* You may suffer with gas, bloating, rumbling and abdominal discomfort. Your stools may be loose, ribbony, pellet-like (rabbit turds) or all of the above. You may be sensitive to certain foods or drinks that didn't bother you before. You shouldn't be losing weight or noticing any blood in your stools. This condition usually improves with time (measured in months), a careful diet, some additional fiber and reassurance. Probiotics (e.g., acidophyllus) may also help. Other gastrointestinal infections and conditions must be ruled out before arriving at this diagnosis. An occasional few unfortunate travelers never return to the way it was before.

The treatment of your diarrhea will again depend upon the cause. But I might be tempted to treat a case of dysentery with an antibiotic (Cipro®, Zithromax®) without waiting for the stool culture, or even a presumptive case of giardiasis with metronidazole (Flagyl®) without awaiting the report on parasites. Hopefully, you have returned home with your bowels intact and that a slight or not so slight case of the runs hasn't dampened your love of travel.

WORMS

This can be an exciting event — almost as exciting as that first view of Machu Picchu or the Taj Majal! But if you happened while abroad to ingest some food that had been contaminated with human feces, or perhaps you didn't cook your beef, pork or fish adequately, then you might have been playing host to a worm for some time. While a bit alarming, this is not usually life-threatening.

Unlike viruses, bacteria and protozoa, worms do not divide inside humans (with the odd exception) so you are unlikely to develop other symptoms. As well, some will not be contagious as they need to spend time incubating in the soil or in an intermediate host like the pig, cow or fish.

There are only four worms capable of being passed in your stools, and the doctor may be able to guess which one it was just by getting a description of the worm and asking where you have been and what you have eaten.

ROUNDWORM (ASCARIS LUMBRICOIDES)

This worm is round, whitish and up to six inches long. It often crawls out into the world because it is having trouble finding a sexual partner inside. Little does it know that it won't find one outside either. The likelihood of acquiring this parasite seems to be inversely proportional to one's budget while away. As most people don't harbor very many worms, there may be no other symptoms. Young children in the tropics who are exposed to contaminated food and water day after day will have lots of worms, stomach aches and distended abdomens. Occasionally a roundworm can get stuck in a small place like your appendix or bile duct and cause more serious problems.

WHIPWORM (TRICHURIS TRICHIURA)

This worm is smaller (3–5 cm) than *Ascaris* and is rarely found in the stools. It is shaped like a whip as its name implies.

PINWORM (ENTEROBIUS VERMICULARIS)

The pinworm (8–13 mm long) can often be seen wandering around your rear end, usually late at night. This is when the female pinworm comes out of the bowel to lay her eggs. The eggs they lay on the skin are quite irritating, typically prompting the infectee (usually a child) to scratch, get the eggs on a couple of fingers, put those fingers in the mouth (or on a little brother) and keep the whole cycle alive. This is not really a tropical or traveler's infection. Rather, it affects close-knit families in temperate climates who pass the sticky eggs back and forth!

The above three infections can be treated with "antihelminthics" such as mebendazole (Vermox®) or albendazole.

TAPEWORM

Worms such as *Taenia saginata* (from uncooked beef), *Taenia solium* (from uncooked pork) and *Diphyllobothrium latum* (from uncooked fish) are the ones that can grow up to 30 feet in length, but usually only short, flat, ribbony segments are passed at one time. Contrary to popular belief, tapeworms are probably not responsible for your weight loss. If you would like to avoid one of these worms, make sure your meat is cooked — well cooked! The treatment of choice for tapeworms is the drug Praziquantel®.

Hopefully, you have captured the worm so it can be identified by your doctor, the lab or even yourself! If not, your stools can be checked (again, poop in the little bottle) for adult worms or the eggs they produce. In the case of pinworms, they are found by doing a "sticky-tape test," that is, applying a sticky little paddle to the skin around the rectum, preferably at night! More than one test may need to be done to detect infection.

SKIN PROBLEMS

BITES

There are many interesting skin conditions that people discover on their return home, but perhaps the most common are nonspecific (we're not really sure what bit you) bites. Mites, bedbugs, fleas, no-see-ums, mosquitoes and many other insects may be responsible. Most of these result in a rash that can be quite itchy. The problem may persist for some time after your return, even though the bugs have been left far behind. This may be due to an allergy or hypersensitivity to the bite itself. Other bites, such as those from the deerfly, tsetse fly or blackfly are usually quite uncomfortable. The treatment of bites might include cool compresses, calamine lotion, topical steroids, antihistamines if you are itchy and antibiotics if they appear infected.

BOILS

Boils can sometimes be large and painful and can be a common problem in travelers. A moist climate, an abundance of bacteria such as *Staphylococcus* and *Streptococcus* and perhaps a relative lack of hygiene may all be responsible. Boils tend to be recurrent and show up over different parts of the body. This is because it is very easy to "inoculate" oneself, simply by touching the infection and then scratching somewhere else. In addition, some people become nasal carriers of the bacteria, and let's face it, most of us get our fingers near our nose on a regular basis. The treatment of an acute boil may be warm saltwater compresses and antibiotics, but an incision to release the pus inside is often required. A longer course of oral antibiotics such as cloxacillin, erythromycin or cephalexin, combined with a topical antibiotic in the nose, may be needed to prevent recurrences.

MYIASIS

Boils may sometimes be confused with myiasis, which is caused by the larva of the botfly, either *Dermatobia hominis* or *Cordylobia anthropophaga*. These flies manage to get their eggs under your skin, either via the bite of a mosquito or by laying them on your clothing, from which they can penetrate your unbroken skin. Most of the travelers I have seen with this condition have just returned from the rain forests of Central America. People with a botfly have the sensation, often a painful one, that there is something alive and moving under their skin, and indeed there is.

The developing larva requires air to survive, and the best way to entice him or her out is to cut off the air supply. This can be accomplished in a few ways, such as cover the little opening with Vaseline®, toothpaste or even raw bacon. Hopefully it will crawl out and you can extract it with a pair of tweezers. If push comes to shove, just applying pressure (lots of pressure) might pop it out. Minor surgery is not usually the way to go. If you are living in the tropics, you may find your pet dog, cat or cattle complaining of the same thing.

CHIGGERS

This problem is caused by infestation with the larvae of the harvest mite, *Trombicula alfreddugesi*, which lives in grass. These critters prefer to be where they are a bit confined, such as around the ankles under a sock or around the beltline. They don't really bite you or suck your blood. Rather they inject an enzyme under the skin. Intense itching occurs at this site, and an allergic reaction can occur, spreading the rash. It may last for weeks. Treatment consists of anti-itch remedies, such as cool compresses or baths, antihistamines and topical steroid creams.

CUTANEOUS LARVA MIGRANS

For the traveler who has just returned from the beaches of Jamaica, Barbados, or in fact any beach and has a creeping, itchy linear rash on the foot, this is undoubtedly cutaneous larva migrans, or a "creeping eruption." The eruption may appear anywhere else on the body, depending upon which part of the anatomy was lying on the sand. It is caused by the larvae of a dog or cat hookworm (*Ancylostoma braziliense* or *Ancylostoma caninum*), which have been left in the sand by the local dog or cat. These larvae can penetrate your unbroken skin, and once having done so they wander aimlessly, in a very serpiginous (winding) pattern under the skin. The red line is intensely itchy, it may blister, and it advances up to an inch per day. It will not enter any vital organs, nor is it transmissible from person to person. While this rash will usually be evident before the end of your vacation, I have seen it appear many months after a return from the tropics. This infection is treated with medications such as albendazole and ivermectin. Freezing and burning are old treatments and somewhat barbaric!

CUTANEOUS LEISHMANIASIS

This is a parasitic disease transmitted by sandflies in many parts of the tropics, particularly the Middle East, Asia and South America. If you have a skin ulcer that just won't heal, this could be what you have.

ESCHAR

An eschar is an easily recognizable skin lesion (by someone who can easily recognize it) left by the bite of a mite or tick. It begins as a small red bump, but gradually turns into a black, crusted ulcer. It is associated with infections such as African tick typhus and scrub typhus. If you have just returned from the game parks in southern Africa with a fever and an odd-looking ulcer on your skin, suggest this diagnosis to your doctor.

LEPROSY

Leprosy still exists in many parts of the world. It is caused by *Mycobacterium leprae*, which is most likely transmitted from person to person via nasal secretions. It's not spread by simply touching an infected person. The skin lesions of leprosy do not look particularly ominous. However, they are usually "numb," or anesthetic, because the underlying nerve is also affected. Leprosy also affects much larger nerves, such as those to the hand and foot, and it is the involvement of these nerves which ultimately leads to the horrible deformities that are often seen with untreated cases. I mention this disease mainly to make you aware that it still exists around the world, but it is not, I repeat not, a risk to travelers.

PHYTOPHOTODERMATITIS

An interesting, though harmless, condition called phyto-photodermatitis occurs in people who have chosen to lighten their hair with lime juice. The juice drips onto the shoulders or face, or it may be rubbed onto other parts of the body after a squeeze of lime into a gin and tonic. The lime reacts with the sunlight, and the result is a streaky, pigmented rash, almost like a mild burn. Fortunately, it fades with time.

RASH

A generalized rash might also be a sign of an infection such as dengue or meningococcal disease, but in this case you would expect to be ill with a fever.

There are many other skin conditions with which you may return, from jock itch (a fungus in your groin) to sporotrichosis. I have discussed the most common ones. And, as I've said repeatedly, it may take the experienced tropical disease doctor to recognize some of these interesting rashes. So if it isn't going away, look for the right help.

PART 4

APPENDIX OF INFECTIOUS DISEASES & CONDITIONS

I have written about malaria, Traveler's Diarrhea and STIs separately, since they are perhaps the most important or common infections encountered by travelers. What follows is a description of "all the rest" — sort of an encyclopedia of exotic and not so exotic infectious diseases and conditions. Some are mentioned in other parts of the book as well. The following list is far from complete, but I have tried to include anything that you may encounter in your travels, your readings or your dinnertime conversations. The conditions below are listed in alphabetical order, not in order of severity.

AMEBIASIS

Entameba histolytica is a protozoal infection of the large bowel that is transmitted through infected food and water. It may cause anything from mild diarrhea to dysentery. Sometimes it causes no symptoms at all. Amebiasis is a parasite with the ability to spread beyond the bowel to other organs such as the skin, the brain and, most often, the liver. An abscess in the liver will cause fever, weight loss and pain in the right upper part of your abdomen. Amebiasis is treated with medications such as metronidazole or tinidazole. A second medication is usually used to eradicate the asymptomatic cysts in the bowel. While it is sometimes diagnosed in travelers, it is probably not very common in reality.

There are a few other amebas — *Entameba coli, Dientameba fragilis, Endolimax nana* and *Entameba hartmanni* that are commonly found in the stools of both travelers and non-travelers. They are considered non-pathogenic; that is, they probably don't cause any serious illness.

ANTHRAX

Anthrax, which had its 15 minutes of fame after 9/11, is caused by the bacterium *Bacillus anthracis*. While mainly an infection of animals (cattle, sheep, goats), humans occasionally get infected if exposed to infected animals or their tissues. Anthrax can affect the skin, lungs or intestines and, in the latter two, can prove fatal. Treatment is with antibiotics such as ciprofloxacin, penicillin or tetracycline.

ASCARIASIS

This is caused by the intestinal roundworm *Ascaris lumbricoides*, which is passed through infected food and water. In areas where human fertilizer is used, it is a great risk. After ingestion, the eggs take a convoluted migration through the veins, the heart, the lungs and back to the intestine. This process takes about 10 to 12 weeks. Remember that almost all worms do not divide in humans, so most travelers who have light exposure will likely have no symptoms. The exception is when an adult worm, often a lonely, solitary worm, starts to migrate, most often out of your rectum. It may also get stuck in small places like the appendix and bile duct. It is easily treatable with medications such as mebendazole and albendazole.

BOILS

In hot, humid climates where bacteria abound and personal hygiene sometimes suffers, small, superficial skin infections sometimes turn into large, painful boils. These may get better with salty soaks or antibiotics, but will sometimes need to be incised. So, be proactive about your cleanliness and treat skin infections early with antiseptics and topical antibiotics.

CAMPYLOBACTER

This bacterial infection with *Campylobacter jejeuni* is a common cause of diarrhea both in travelers and back home.

It is particularly prevalent in Southeast Asia, where it is also resistant to the antibiotic Cipro®. It is transmitted by eating undercooked food or unpasteurized dairy products. Undercooked poultry is particularly dangerous. After a brief incubation period of two to five days, you may develop fever and chills, followed by lower abdominal cramps and diarrhea. Blood and mucus may be present in the stools. The diagnosis is made by doing a stool culture, something that is unlikely to occur on your trip abroad. While the infection will resolve on its own, antibiotics such as Cipro® and Zithromax® will shorten its duration.

CHAGAS DISEASE

Chagas disease, or American trypanosomiasis, is a protozoal infection and disease of poverty that still occurs in rural Central and South America. It is passed on by a particularly disgusting bug known as the reduviid bug, which lives in the cracked walls of mud and adobe huts and thatched roofs. There is also the danger of transmission via blood transfusions. The infection is usually transmitted at night, when the bug feeds on its host and, in fact, defecates around the eye.

Early symptoms may include swelling around the eye and flu-like symptoms. Many years later, the symptoms of chronic infection may appear; these consist of a gross enlargement of the heart, the esophagus and the bowel. This infection is rare in travelers, but if you find yourself sleeping in the type of housing I described, sleep under an insect net.

CHIKUNGUNYA VIRUS

Perhaps the most exotic-sounding infection we have, Chikungunya is an emerging infection in Asia and Africa. Along with dengue fever, it is affectionately known as "monsoon fever" in India, where huge outbreaks have occurred. *Aedes aegypti*, the same mosquito that transmits dengue fever, and *Aedes albopicutus* are the main vectors. Recall that these are daytime biting mosquitoes that like to breed around human dwellings in small collections of water. Symptoms begin 2 to 12 days after being bitten and include fever, headache, fatigue, nausea, vomiting, muscle pain, rash and joint pain. It may last a few days to a few weeks and resolves without treatment other than analgesics (avoid aspirin). The diagnosis is made by serology or antibody tests, and the virus needs to be differentiated from other febrile illnesses, like dengue fever, malaria and typhoid fever.

CIGUATERA POISONING

This isn't really an infection, but I put it here anyway. This unpleasant condition is caused by the toxin of a tiny organism, *Gambierdiscus toxicus*, which is found along the coral reefs of the Caribbean and South Pacific. This organism is consumed by the local reef fish (barracuda, red snapper, grouper, kingfish, sea bass, Spanish mackerel and surgeonfish), which in turn are eaten by larger and larger fish. The toxin doesn't harm the fish, so they look and smell normal. Cooking or freezing doesn't make a difference.

The symptoms of ciguatera poisoning, which include abdominal cramps, nausea and vomiting, usually begin within 12 hours of eating the guilty fish and may last for one or two days. Other, more interesting symptoms include paresthesias, or numbness, around the mouth and in the extremities, severe itching, weakness and temperature reversal, that is, what is cold feels hot, and vice versa. These symptoms may last for weeks or months.

The diagnosis of ciguatera poisoning is a clinical one, and treatment consists mainly of supportive measures. To avoid this one, either avoid eating reef fish or stick to the smaller fish; and avoid the head and organs, where there is more toxin.

COLD INJURIES

There are many popular destinations where the risk of cold injury exists. Many of these places are literally right in our own backyards. Temperature decreases with altitude, not only leading to cold injury, but also aggravating altitude sickness. Alcohol consumption, cigarette smoking and wearing tight or wet clothing will also add to the risk of such injuries.

Frostbite

Frostbite is what occurs when our body tissues freeze. It is most likely to happen on an exposed surface, such as the ears, the nose or an extremity (the fingers and toes). When freezing occurs, ice crystals form within the cells. Remember that water expands when it freezes to ice, causing the cells to rupture and die. That, along with impairment of the local circulation, leads to death of the tissues.

Frostbite requires rewarming. The tissues should be handled carefully to avoid causing more damage. Bandages and a splint should be applied. The main pitfall in the treatment of frostbite is the danger of refreezing and, hence, more tissue damage. For that reason, rewarming should not be started until you are sure there will be no further exposure to the cold. It's better to hobble on a frostbitten foot until proper medical care is available than to thaw the extremity, only to have it freeze again. It may take several months before the extent of damage from frostbite is evident, but certainly loss of fingers, toes and ears can occur.

Frostnip

Frostnip usually precedes frostbite. At this stage, only the superficial layers of the skin have frozen. This is comparable to a first-degree burn. The affected area will appear white or gray in light-skinned people or pink or red in dark-skinned people and will feel numb. Movement remains intact. If further exposure takes place, it may become blistered and turn black. Frostbite, in contrast, occurs when all of the tissues — skin, nerves, muscles, blood vessels — have frozen. The skin will appear white or bluish, and feel woody to the touch. Movement is lost and sensation is absent.

Frostnip should be treated promptly if possible, as it may continue on to frostbite if left untreated. Immersing the affected part in warm water (105°F/40.5°C) and protecting it from further cold should suffice. If you can't find your thermometer, the water should feel hot, but not too uncomfortable to touch. Warm up your body as well with some hot soup and warm clothing. The rewarming process may be quite uncomfortable, and an analgesic such as aspirin or ibuprofen may be taken.

Chilblains and Trench Foot

These are milder injuries than frostbite, and they occur when an extremity is exposed to both wet and cold. The treatment is similar to that for frostbite, and there are usually no long-term problems.

Hypothermia

When we are exposed to cold environments, the body has two methods of coping. Number one: the blood vessels to the skin constrict or narrow, so that our blood flow is redirected to the center of the body and we lose less heat to the environment. If this doesn't work, number two kicks in: we shiver, which produces heat through muscle action. When these mechanisms are overwhelmed, our core temperature falls below 96°F/35.5°C. This dip may occur quickly, such as when we are dropped in frigid water; or it may happen more gradually, over hours or days. The very old or very young, the intoxicated or those on certain medications may be predisposed to hypothermia.

In addition to being cold and shivering, the hypothermic person may become confused, irritable and, eventually, comatose. This response is not unlike high altitude cerebral edema (HACE), which may be aggravated by hypothermia.

To treat hypothermia:

- Get the person out of the cold, away from the wind and moisture, and off the cold ground.
- Remove any wet or cold clothing.
- Cover the person with warm blankets, a sleeping bag or dry clothing. Apply heat sources, such as a hot water bottle or heating pad (but not directly on the skin).
- Warm up the environment with a fire, some sunshine or warm bodies.
- Don't aim for rapid rewarming (for example, immersing the person in warm water).
- Offer warm fluids and something sweet to eat.

More severe hypothermia is a medical emergency and requires transport to a medical facility.

CRYPTOSPORIDIOSIS

This protozoal infection is an uncommon cause of Traveler's Diarrhea. It typically causes watery diarrhea that may last for up to three weeks. In patients who are immunosuppressed with HIV/AIDS, it can be particularly lethal. Treatment consists mainly of rehydration as there is no real effective medication for this infection. Iodine may not kill the organism, so drinking water should be boiled or treated with chlorine dioxide (Pristine®).

CUTANEOUS LARVA MIGRANS

This infection causes one of the more interesting rashes in returning travelers. People walking or lying on the beach may unwittingly be penetrated by this microscopic dog or cat hookworm. Being in the wrong host, it wanders aimlessly in a winding path, usually on the foot but occasionally on the butt or breast depending on how you were lying. The rash is very itchy and often blisters. It is not contagious to others and will not crawl into more important organs. The diagnosis is made by recognizing it, and it should be treated with oral albendazole, as opposed to burning or freezing. I have seen it most often in travelers from Barbados and Jamaica, but it can happen on any dog-frequented beach.

DENGUE FEVER

This viral infection belongs to the same family as yellow fever, West Nile virus and Japanese encephalitis. It is transmitted by the *Aedes* mosquito, which likes to breed in small collections of water, such as those found in or around tires, planters, vases and construction sites. That makes it a peridomestic mosquito that is found in urban areas. Unlike the *Anopheles* vector of malaria, it is a daytime biter. The infection may be seasonal, being most prevalent during and after the rainy season. Dengue is on the rise for several reasons including urban migration, poverty, smart mosquitoes and perhaps global warming. (In India it is known as monsoon fever.)

After a short incubation period of between five and eight days, the illness begins abruptly with a high fever, severe headache (behind the eyes) and severe pains in the bones. A fine rash may appear after a few days. There are four strains of dengue, and those who are exposed to a subsequent strain, usually children living in less developed countries, may develop dengue hemorrhagic fever, a much more serious illness. Spontaneous bleeding may occur, the blood pressure drops and it may prove fatal. The treatment of dengue is supportive, i.e., analgesics, fluids and blood products to stop any bleeding.

For the traveler, prevention involves using effective insect repellents during the day, and for those who are living there, getting rid of potential breeding sites around the home. Vaccines against dengue are in development, but who knows when they will be available.

FILARIASIS

Filariasis, caused by the tiny roundworms *Wuchereria bancrofti* and *Brugia malayi*, is transmitted by mosquitoes throughout most of the tropics. These worms find their way into your lymph nodes and vessels, usually in the groin. The initial symptoms, which don't occur until at least three months after infection, include fever and inflammation of the lymph nodes. With chronic and repeated infections, the lymph tracts become obstructed. The obstruction in turn may cause chronic swelling of the leg or foot, as well as fairly grotesque changes to the skin. It is a major cause of disability and disfigurement in the tropics. This condition is better known as elephantiasis, as it is an elephant's foot which it most resembles. The infection is quite rare in travelers. It is diagnosed by finding the microfilaria or larvae in the blood (interestingly, they are mainly found at night) and by antibody tests. Treatment is with medications such as albendazole, ivermectin and diethylcarbamazine. This is a rare infection in travelers.

GIARDIASIS

This infection of the small intestine is caused by the almost "human-looking" protozoa *Giardia lamblia*. It is the most common intestinal parasite in travelers. It is found world-wide, and is sometimes called "beaver fever" (it does not cause a fever). Infection follows ingestion of the cysts of the parasite in contaminated food and water.

The incubation period is longer than for bacteria, being about two weeks. Symptoms may vary from nothing at all, to mild or severe diarrhea. There should be no blood or mucus in the stools. This is usually accompanied by other symptoms such as loss of appetite, fatigue, nausea, gas and bloating. Farts that "curl your nose" have been described. Weight loss may occur due to malabsorption of nutrients. Lactose intolerance is common. This infection should be suspected when your diarrhea has gone on for a few weeks.

Giardiasis is diagnosed by finding the characteristic parasite in a stool sample. As well, several commercially available tests to detect *Giardia* antigen in the stool exist. Treatment consists of a course of metronidazole, or tinidazole, if it is available.

HEAT EXPOSURE

When your car's cooling mechanism breaks down, things go terribly wrong. Smoke starts coming out from under the hood and four-letter words start coming out of your mouth. Our body is no different. We have two main mechanisms to keep our core temperature at about 98.6°F/37°C in the face of extreme heat. First, our blood is redirected to the skin and our blood vessels dilate. This allows us to radiate some of the excess heat into the environment. Then we sweat — hopefully a lot. As the sweat evaporates, it acts to cool us down. When the humidity is high, the sweat may not evaporate as quickly or at all. In very dry or windy conditions, it may evaporate so quickly that you don't even notice yourself dripping. Your ability to adapt may also depend on your age and certain medications that you may be taking.

Heat exhaustion

Exhaustion is the first sign of trouble. It is characterized by a normal or slightly elevated temperature, headache, thirst, nausea and vomiting, dizziness and weakness and, as the name implies, exhaustion. The skin may be pale, cool or moist.

To treat heat exhaustion:

- Move the person into a cooler spot, such as the shade (most sensible local people are already there). Remove excess clothing.
- Replace fluids. Oral rehydration will usually suffice (the cooler the better). Drink small amounts of fluid frequently, rather than gulping down large amounts, which may result in further vomiting. Keep track of urine output to assess the state of hydration. Clear urine is better than dark, concentrated urine.

Heatstroke

True heatstroke is a medical emergency. The body's cooling mechanisms have failed. The temperature rises dramatically, often as high as 106°F/41°C. The skin is red, hot and dry. Confusion may progress to loss of consciousness. Your initial treatment may involve cooling the person with cool, wet towels or sheets, ice packs and fanning. Seeking out more sophisticated medical care is necessary.

Prickly heat

Prickly heat, or heat rash, is not quite a life-threatening condition, but it can be a nuisance and it is common in hot, humid climates. It is caused when the narrow ducts through which sweat travels to the surface become clogged. This results in itching, irritation and small blisters or red bumps, mainly on the trunk and the thighs. Treatment consists of somehow keeping your skin cool and dry, and perhaps applying a cortisone cream.

HEPATITIS – VIRAL

Hepatitis means "itis" or inflammation of the "hepar" or liver — that large organ located under your right ribcage. Several viruses can cause this, including hepatitis A through E. Symptoms of hepatitis, regardless of which virus is causing it, consist of fever, fatigue, loss of appetite, nausea, pain around the liver, itchiness and jaundice (yellowing of the skin and eyes). **Hepatitis A and B** are vaccine-preventable infections. **Hepatitis C** is very similar to hepatitis B. It is transmitted in the same way and it may lead to chronic liver disease. **Hepatitis E** resembles hepatitis A; however, it may be more serious in pregnant women, sometimes leading to liver failure, premature delivery or spontaneous abortion. No vaccines are available for these two infections (C and E).

LEISHMANIASIS

There are several strains of this protozoal infection, some of which affect the skin (cutaneous leishmaniasis) and others which affect the internal organs like the liver and spleen (visceral leishmaniasis). It is transmitted by sandflies. The cutaneous form is found in the rain forests of Central and South America, the deserts of Asia and in the Middle East. Archaeologists hunting through rubble and soldiers in Iraq are among those travelers who get infected. The ulcers it causes are typically found on the face or extremities, and will eventually heal with scarring. Certain strains may spread to the cartilage of the nose or throat and cause horrible deformity. Visceral leishmaniasis, or kala azar, occurs mainly in India, Bangladesh, Nepal, Sudan and Brazil and causes massive enlargement of the liver and spleen and severe anemia. Without treatment, it is usually fatal. This one is another rarity in travelers.

LEPTOSPIROSIS

This potentially fatal infection is caused by the spirochete *Leptospira interrogans*, which is primarily an infection of animals, such as rats, mice, dogs and farm animals. Humans become infected when they become contaminated with urine from infected animals. This may happen through accidental ingestion or penetration of broken skin or mucus membranes (around the eyes). This would imply that people end up in the same freshwater lakes and streams where these animals pee. While an unusual infection in travelers, it has occurred in outbreaks, such as the Eco-Challenge in Sabah in the year 2000.

After an incubation period of between 2 and 21 days, you may experience fever, headache, chills, muscle aches, vomiting, diarrhea and red eyes. Most of this sounds like malaria or other febrile illnesses. Most infections will be mild and resolve on their own. In more serious cases, the brain, liver or kidney may be affected. The diagnosis is made by serological testing, and it is treated with antibiotics such as doxycycline, azithromycin or penicillin. For high-risk travelers, that is those who must spend time in urine-infected waters (perhaps after flooding), prophylactic doxycycline (200 mg/week) can be used.

LOA LOA

This filarial infection is found mainly in the tropical forests of West Africa and is passed by the fly *Chrysops*. The 3 cm long worm crawls under the skin, causing a moving swelling known as a Calabar swelling, named after a city in Nigeria.

Much more exciting is when the worm wanders across the eye. Treatment is with the drug diethylcarbamazine. You are very, very unlikely to catch this one.

MYIASIS

This one is a bit disgusting. Myiasis is an infection of the skin caused by the larvae of certain flies that are present in the tropics. The two main species are *Dermatobia hominis* (the human botfly) in South and Central America, and *Cordylobia anthropophaga* in Africa. Both of these can also infect animals such as cattle, dogs and cats. Most of the infections I've seen have been in travelers visiting the rain forests of Costa Rica and Belize.

The eggs of the fly manage to get attached to the underside of a female mosquito and penetrate the unbroken skin when the mosquito feeds. It may also be possible for these eggs to be deposited on clothing or towels left out to dry, and then rubbed into the skin. At the site of penetration, a boil-like lesion develops fairly rapidly. It will be red and tender. People often complain of transient, shooting pains in the lesion, as if there is something moving inside. There is! A tiny opening is usually visible at the top, through which the little maggot gets his or her air.

Getting rid of these things is the most fun. While it is always tempting to make a small incision and cut it out, this is not usually the wisest decision. There are better ways to entice the little critter out, and most of these ways involve suffocation. Try closing the little air hole with Vaseline, toothpaste or raw bacon overnight, and you may see him or her wriggling at the opening in the morning. It can then be grasped with tweezers and gently extricated. Peanut butter, toothpaste or chewing tobacco may also work. Patience is a virtue. When all else fails, good old squeezing, hopefully with an anesthetic, will do the trick.

Don't spend your time worrying about this one. But use your insect repellents, shake out your towels and iron your clothing. And if you do end up with one of these things, take it out and send it to me. I must tell you that one of the readers of my first book diagnosed it herself and embarrassed her dermatologist.

NOROVIRUS (NORWALK VIRUS)

This viral infection is one of the few for which cruisers are at greater risk. It is extremely infectious and is contracted through contaminated food and water, from close contact with infected individuals and even from handling infected surfaces such as doorknobs. Most people recover after about three days of intense nausea, vomiting and watery diarrhea. The treatment is fluid replacement. Prevention consists of washing your hands, washing your hands and avoiding sick people. The more paranoid may wish to disinfect their telephones, doorknobs and barbells.

ONCHOCERCIASIS

River blindness, as this infection is commonly known, is caused by a filarial worm that is transmitted by the bite of blackflies. Most cases occur in remote African rural agricultural villages, located near rapidly flowing streams, but it is also found in Latin America and Yemen. It is highly unlikely to be a risk to travelers, unless they are living or working along such streams for long periods of time. There are three main symptoms — nodules under the skin that contain the adult worms, an itchy rash and eye lesions which can lead to blindness. It is diagnosed by a skin biopsy or "skin snip," and treatment is with the drug ivermectin. If you think you are at risk, then wear long clothing and use insect repellents.

RIFT VALLEY FEVER

This viral infection is a major killer of livestock but can infect humans who are in contact with infected animals. It may also be transmitted by mosquitoes and by drinking the unpasteurized milk of these animals. As its name suggests, it occurs mainly in the Rift Valley of Africa, though it has popped up in the Middle East. After an incubation period of two to six days, it usually causes a mild flu-like illness and most will recover within a week. However more serious forms may cause bleeding, or involve the liver, brain or eyes.

SALMONELLA

This is a food- and water-borne infection caused by numerous strains of the bacterium *Salmonella*. The incubation period is between 12 and 72 hours, and diarrhea usually last between four and seven days. Dysentery with fever and blood and pus in the stools may occur. In the young, the old and the immunosuppressed, the infection may spread to the bloodstream causing serious illness. It is diagnosed by stool culture, and can be treated with fluid replacement and antibiotics such as Cipro® or Zithromax®. A small percentage of patients will continue to harbor the bacteria after recovery, as did Typhoid Mary. This state may be eradicated with antibiotics or by removing the gall bladder.

SCHISTOSOMIASIS

This disease of poverty affects more than 200 million people throughout the tropics. It is caused by a tiny worm whose eggs are passed by humans in the urine or feces, depending on the species (there are three). The eggs invade the local snails, and eventually emerge back into the fresh water and penetrate the unbroken skin of children playing or women washing in the infected water. After a migration through the heart and lungs, the adult worms settle in the veins of the bladder or bowel, have sex and produce eggs. It is the eggs that damage the bowel and liver, and the bladder and kidneys. Children, who have the most freshwater exposure suffer the most.

Travelers are at risk when they swim in Lake Malawi, fall out of their boats on the Zambezi or get exposed in other bodies of fresh water. Again, considering that worms don't divide in their human hosts, most infected travelers will not suffer significant disease. The diagnosis is made by finding the characteristic eggs in the urine or stools, or through antibody testing. Treatment is with praziquantel, and many people who have been exposed choose to treat themselves before leaving Africa.

SHIGELLA

This bacterium causes perhaps the most severe form of Traveler's Diarrhea. Bacillary dysentery, with fever, chills, and blood and pus in the stools is common. It is diagnosed by stool culture (which is unlikely to be done in the middle of India). Most intestinal bacterial infections have a fairly short incubation period, that is, it doesn't take long to get sick after ingesting the offending food. This is when you would really like to have an antibiotic such as Cipro® or Zithromax® handy.

SLEEPING SICKNESS

This does not refer to people with insomnia, but rather, it is a protozoan infection (*Trypanosoma gambiense* or *rhodiense*) passed by tsetse flies in sub-Saharan Africa. Initial symptoms consist of a painful sore at the site of the bite, fever, swollen glands, headache and insomnia. In the later stages, six to nine months later, irritability, drowsiness by day and insomnia by night may occur. Mental functions decline and death eventually occurs from malnutrition or other infections. This infection is extremely rare in travelers, but if out on safari, why not cover up anyway.

TAPEWORMS

Aside from the shock of learning that these can be as long as 30 feet, they usually don't cause much problem. The main symptom is usually passing a small, flat, ribbony segment of the worm in the stool. They are acquired by eating beef (*Taenia saginata*), pork (*Taenia solium*) or fish (*Diphyllobothrium latum*) that has been inadequately cooked. The myth that people who can't gain weight have a tapeworm is just that. The pork tapeworm has the ability to spread to the brain and cause seizures, and can be infectious to others. It is diagnosed by identifying the segments or the eggs in the stools. Treatment is with praziquantel.

TICK TYPHUS

Ticks transmit more than 25 different infections worldwide. Just like ice cream, ticks come in hard and soft. Forms of tick typhus come in many varieties — African, Indian, Mediterranean, Australian and Israeli. I have seen it mainly in people returning from South African game parks. The infectious organism is a type of bacterium known as *Rickettsia*. After an incubation period of one to two weeks, one develops fever, headache, swollen glands near the bite, an eschar (a black, crusted skin lesion) and a rash. It is diagnosed on clinical suspicion and antibody tests. Malaria must also be considered. Treatment is with doxycycline. To avoid this and a myriad of other tick-borne diseases, cover up with long sleeves and pants, use insect repellent, and do a "tick check" at the end of the day. They can be easily removed by applying gentle traction with a pair of tweezers.

VIRAL HEMORRHAGIC FEVERS (VHFs)

This is a scary group of viruses which normally infects small mammals such as rats and mice, and humans become accidental victims. The best known of these viral illnesses are Lassa fever, Ebola hemorrhagic fever and Marburg hemorrhagic fever, all of which occur sporadically in sub-Saharan Africa. Hantavirus pulmonary syndrome is found in the western hemisphere, including North America while Crimean-Congo hemorrhagic fever can be found in Africa, Asia and Europe. Human infection occurs when we become contaminated with the urine, feces or saliva of the actual host. Once infected, human to human transmission can occur through medical care or sex.

VHFs may seem like flu, malaria or typhoid, but can become complicated by internal bleeding and lung, liver or kidney failure. Treatment is mainly supportive, though the drug Ribavirin® is used to treat Lassa fever. Mortality rates range from about 15 percent to more than 50 percent with Ebola. If you develop a flu-like illness while away, this one goes at the bottom of your worry list, unless you happen to be the doctor tending to the local outbreak.

FURTHER READING

International Organizations and Medical Sites:

Centers for Disease Control and Prevention (CDC): www.cdc.gov/travel

Public Health Agency of Canada (PHAC): www.phac-aspc.gc.ca/tmp-pmv/index-eng.php

World Health Organization (WHO): www.who.int

Pan American Health Organization (PAHO): http://new.paho.org

International Society of Travel Medicine (ISTM): www.istm.org

CIWEC Clinic (Travel Medicine Center), Kathmandu, Nepal: http://ciwec-clinic.com

International Association for Medical Assistance to Travelers (IAMAT): www.iamat.org

Department of Foreign Affairs and Trade (Canada): www.voyage.gc.ca

U.S. Department of State — International Travel: http://travel.state.gov/travel/travel_1744.html

High Altitude Medical Guide: www.high-altitude-medicine.com

The Travel Clinic: www.drwisetravel.com

The Mayo Clinic — First Aid: www.mayoclinic.com/health/FirstAidIndex/FirstAidIndex

Helpful Travel Sites

Journeywoman: www.journeywoman.com

Lonely Planet: www.lonelyplanet.com

Verge Magazine: www.vergemagazine.com

National Geographic: www.nationalgeographic.com

Perry-Castañeda Library Map Collection: www.lib.utexas.edu/maps/index.html

Society for Accessible Travel and Hospitality (SATH): www.sath.org

Universal Currency Converter: www.xe.net/ucc

International weather: www.wxusa.com/international/B.htm

References in Print and Enjoyable Reading

Auerbach, P.S. 2009. *Medicine for the Outdoors*. 5th ed. Maryland Heights, MO: Elsevier.

Gallmann, Kuki. 1991. *I Dreamed of Africa*. New York: Penguin.

Herzog, Maurice. 1953. *Annapurna*. New York: Dutton.

Journal of Travel Medicine. Hoboken, NJ: Wiley-Blackwell. (See also website listed above.)

Keystone, Jay S. et al, eds. 2008. *Travel Medicine*. 2d ed. Maryland Heights, MO: Elsevier.

Krakauer, Jon. 1997. *Into Thin Air*. New York: Random House.

Ondaatje, Christopher. 1998. *Journey to the Source of the Nile*. Toronto: HarperCollins.

Preston, Richard M. 1994. *The Hot Zone*. New York: Doubleday.

Theroux, Paul. 2003. *Dark Star Safari: Overland from Cairo to Cape Town*. New York: Houghton Mifflin.

Werner, David. 1992. *Where There Is No Doctor*. 2d ed (updated 2009). Berkeley, CA: Hesperian Foundation.

INDEX

176

177

78

globulin), 28
Humira, 40
hypothermia, 159–60
hypoxia, 72

I

IAMAT, 54
immune modulators, 40
immunosuppression, 15, 19,
   23, 39–41. *See also* HIV/
   AIDS
Imodium (loperamide), 42,
   83–84
Imovax, 27
India, 81, 121
infants, 15, 60, 68, 106
infections, 13–14. *See also*
   specific diseases
inflammatory bowel disease
   (IBD), 38
influenza, 16–17, 41
INH (isoniazid), 31
inoculations. *See* vaccinations
insects, 104–7. *See also*
   specific types
   repellents, 42, 69, 105–7
insurance, 52–54, 98
International Association
   for Medical Assistance to
   Travellers (IAMAT), 54
iodine, 82
irritable bowel syndrome
   (post-infectious), 142–43
isoniazid (INH), 31
Ivory Coast, 19
Ixiaro, 26

J

Japanese encephalitis, 25–26,
   107
jaundice, yellow. *See* hepatitis
   A
jellyfish, 114–15

jet lag, 62–66
jock itch, 151

K

kala azar, 165–66
The Keeper, 45
Keystone, Jay, 49

L

lactose intolerance, 79, 80,
   141, 142, 163
Lariam (mefloquine), 125–26
larva migrans, cutaneous, 149,
   161
Lassa fever, 172
Latin America, 81. *See also*
   specific countries
leishmaniasis, 107, 149,
   165–66
lemon eucalyptus insect
   repellents, 107
leprosy, 150
leptospirosis, 137, 166
Liberia, 19
lice, 107
loa loa, 107, 166–67
loperamide (Imodium), 42,
   83–84
lung disease, 35, 38–39, 76
Lyme disease, 107

M

Machu Picchu, 74
malaria, 118–31. *See also*
   antimalarials
   cause, 118–19
   cerebral, 119, 120, 136
   chloroquine and, 139–40
   diagnosis, 128–29
   locations, 121–22
   myths about, 129–30
   Plasmodium falciparum,

183

184

19–20, 40
immunosuppression and,
15, 19, 23, 39–40
pain minimizing, 47
pregnancy and, 15, 16, 19,
23, 26, 29, 42
proof of, 17–19
recommended, 19, 20–31
required, 17–20
routine, 15–17
side effects, 20, 32
vaginal infections, 45
valuables, 93
Vanuatu, 121
Vaqta, 21
varicella (chicken pox), 15
Verorab, 27
VHFs (viral hemorrhagic
fevers), 172
Vibramycin (doxycycline), 127
Vibrio cholera, 80
violence, 92–95
viruses, 80. *See also specific
diseases*
visiting friends and relatives
(VFRs), 49–50
Vivaxim, 21, 23
Vivotif, 23

W

Waddell, Chris, 37
water
drinking, 82
immersion in, 170
West Nile virus, 107
whipworm (*Trichuris
trichiura*), 145
women, 43–45, 99, 126
worms (intestinal), 80, 144–46

X

Xifaxan (rifaximin), 38, 41,
83, 84

Y

yeast infections, 45, 127
YEL-AVD (yellow fever
vaccine-associated
viscerotropic disease), 20
yellow fever, 17–20, 107
yellow jaundice. *See* hepatitis A

Z

zanamivir (Relenza), 17
zinc oxide, 69
Zithromax (azithromycin), 38,
42, 47, 84
Zofran, 76
zolpidem, 65
zopiclone, 65

185

ACKNOWLEDGMENTS

I owe a great debt of gratitude to my family — Gayle, Carrie, Adam and Hannah, Benjamin and Ros and Michael — for supporting me and putting up with me and traveling with me. My office staff, Indi, Demi, Karon and Eve, help to make my work life enjoyable. There are several friends — they know who they are — whom I thank as always for their friendship. And finally my Dad, Sydney, who again has caught all of my spelling and grammatical errors just in time!

NOTES

NOTES

NOTES

NOTES